Fundamentals of
Epidemiology and Biostatistics

Fundamentals of
Epidemiology and Biostatistics

Shyam Sunder Deepti

MD (Community Medicine), MA (Sociology), MSc (Applied Psychology)

Associate Professor and Head
Department of Community Medicine
Government Medical College
Amritsar, Punjab

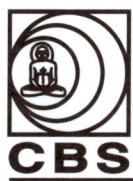

CBS

CBS Publishers & Distributors Pvt Ltd

New Delhi • Bengaluru • Chennai • Kochi • Kolkata • Mumbai
Bhopal • Bhubaneswar • Hyderabad • Jharkhand • Nagpur • Patna • Pune
• Uttarakhand • Dhaka (Bangladesh)

Fundamentals of
Epidemiology and Biostatistics

ISBN: 978-81-239-2584-4

Copyright © Author and Publishers

First Edition: 2014

Reprint: 2019

Published by Satish Kumar Jain and produced by Varun Jain for

CBS Publishers & Distributors Pvt Ltd

4819/XI Prahlad Street, 24 Ansari Road, Daryaganj, New Delhi 110 002, India.
Ph: 23289259, 23266861, 23266867   Website: www.cbspd.com
Fax: 011-23243014   e-mail: delhi@cbspd.com; cbspubs@airtelmail.in.
Corporate Office: 204 FIE, Industrial Area, Patparganj, Delhi 110 092
Ph: 4934 4934   Fax: 4934 4935   e-mail: publishing@cbspd.com; publicity@cbspd.com

Branches

- **Bengaluru:** Seema House 2975, 17th Cross, K.R. Road, Banasankari 2nd Stage, Bengaluru 560 070, Karnataka, India.
  Ph: +91-80-26771678/79   Fax: +91-80-26771680   e-mail: bangalore@cbspd.com
- **Chennai:** 7, Subbaraya Street, Shenoy Nagar, Chennai 600 030, Tamil Nadu, India.
  Ph: +91-44-26680620, 26681266   Fax: +91-44-42032115   e-mail: chennai@cbspd.com
- **Kochi:** 42/1325, 1326, Power House Road, Opp. KSEB Power House, Ernakulam 682 018, Kochi, Kerala, India.
  Ph: +91-484-4059061-65   Fax: +91-484-4059065   e-mail: kochi@cbspd.com
- **Kolkata:** 6/B, Ground Floor, Rameswar Shaw Road, Kolkata-700 014, West Bengal, India.
  Ph: +91-33-22891126, 22891127, 22891128   e-mail: kolkata@cbspd.com
- **Mumbai:** 83-C, Dr E Moses Road, Worli, Mumbai-400018, Maharashtra, India.
  Ph: +91-22-24902340/41   Fax: +91-22-24902342   e-mail: mumbai@cbspd.com

Representatives

• **Bhopal** 0-8319310552	• **Bhubaneswar** 0-9911037372	• **Hyderabad** 0-9885175004	
• **Jharkhand** 0-9811541605	• **Nagpur** 0-9421945513	• **Patna** 0-9334159340	
• **Pune** 0-9623451994	• **Uttarakhand** 0-9716462459	• **Dhaka** 01912-003485 (Bangladesh)	

Printed at India Binding House, Noida, UP, India

to

_____

my better half
Usha Deepti

Foreword

Epidemiological methods play a key role in identifying environmental, social, behavioral and genetic determinants of disease process. Epidemiology and biostatistics are branches of the basic science which quantify the disease process and play a major role in developing and evaluating health policies relating to social/legal issues. A clear understanding of the fundamental aspects of epidemiology and biostatistics is needed to successfully navigate the complex methods utilised in research studies. The medical professionals need to know the basic epidemiological methods covering etiologic as well as prognostic factors of the disease processes so as to conceive policies for better health.

The primary goal of this book, conceived by Dr SS Deepti, a teacher par excellence and genius in writings, is to recreate the perspective of learning epidemiology and biostatistics in a student-friendly manner. The book provides basic principles of epidemiology with many examples of application of epidemiology to public health and clinical practice. The text is written in a very lucid manner so as to have a clear understanding of the subject. The students' queries, which they might have asked in the class, are nicely explained in this book.

The book will be a boon for the medical students as well as health professionals undertaking clinical research studies. I keep this book in a "must-read" category and recommend the same to students, teachers, health workers and anyone associated with effective epidemiological methods.

Vimal K Sikri
Principal
Government Dental College and Hospital
Amristar
and
Director
Punjab Institute of Medical Sciences
Jalandhar

Preface

Man's fight with disease is a continuous process. Since times immemorial, researchers have been finding causes and cure of various diseases inflicting humans. The need to prevent a disease process or at least slow down its effect on living tissues has always been a challenge for medical professionals. The basic rationale is to promote optimal health of the society coupled with minimizing the damage caused by the disease process.

Epidemiology and biostatistics are the branches of basic science which quantify the disease process and play a major role in developing and evaluating health policies relating to social/legal issues. The primary goal of this book is to recreate the perspective of learning epidemiology and biostatistics in a student-friendly manner.

Epidemiologic methods play a key role in identifying environmental, social, behavioral and genetic determinants of disease process. Clinical epidemiology addresses the transmission from onset of disease to health. Descriptive epidemiology provides the disease pattern that is needed to look at health in a broader perspective, subsequently setting the priorities. A clear understanding of the fundamental aspects of epidemiology and biostatistics is needed to successfully navigate the complex methods utilized in research studies. The medical professionals need to know the basic epidemiological methods covering etiologic as well as prognostic factors of the disease processes so as to conceive policies for better health.

The book provides basic principles of epidemiology with many examples of application of epidemiology to public health and clinical practice. The text is written in a very lucid manner so that a reader can have a clear understanding of the subject. The dedicated help of the students in the form of questions they asked in the class is inborn in the book.

The book will be a boon for the medical students as well as the health professionals undertaking clinical research studies.

S S Deepti

Acknowledgement

During my teaching carrier in the subject of community medicine, I always felt that epidemiology is the exclusive trait of expertise. It also fascinated me because of its content as it helps to inculcate scientific attitude in one.

I always prefer to teach epidemiology to my students with the perspective to develop an attitude of 5 Ws (What?, Where?, Who?, When? and Why?).

Medical students have always been repulsive of biostatistics as it was very close to mathematics. But thanks to Mr RL Aggarwal, statistics teacher of my MD classes, who made it easier and interesting. We would correlate it with medical science. Now, I completely believe that epidemiology is incomplete without biostatistics.

Writing has always been my passion and I am a regular writer in Punjabi. This is my first attempt at this level. Although, I have one more book which was the first initiative in the field of practical community medicine which because of various reasons remained confined to the state of Punjab only. Dr AS Padda, former professor and head of department, was an equal participant in the book and I can feel his presence in this book too. I would also like to thank Dr Vimal Sikri, Principal, Government Dental College, Amristar, for his encouraging words about me and this book.

For this initiative I would also like to thank all my colleagues of the department and also my postgraduate students who encouraged and helped me to complete this task with their contribution at various levels.

S S Deepti

Contents

Part 2: **Biostatistics**

PART I

Epidemiology

1

Concept of Epidemiology

INTRODUCTION

Today, when we talk about epidemiology, we mean, 'the science of study of frequency, distribution and determinants of health related states in human population, and the art of application of the results of this study for the control of health problems as described by 'Last' in 1988. Of course, it's a fact that epidemiology took its origin from the word 'epidemic' and it begins with the study of outbreak of epidemics (1873) like cholera, plague, etc. In 1927 when non-communicable diseases or better named as life-style diseases replaced the communicable diseases in frequency and magnitude, the scope of epidemiology widened. Due to its various study designs, the concept of epidemiology has gone further to involve, not only disease situations but physiological and other health related states as mother and child health, drug addiction, etc. Furthermore, evaluating the health care delivery of the community and treatment regimes, newer areas of concern like health planning, primary health care interventions like vitamin A supplementation, immunization, etc. have also emerged.

In 1873, Parkin defined it as a branch of medical science which treats epidemics. After that, additions and alternations were made and ultimately WHO accepted the definition given by 'Last' in 1988.

As a member of modern scientific principle, we can use these words, like reliability, validity, accuracy, sensitivity and specificity with confidence, because our discipline is based on epidemiology. In fact epidemiology is the only discipline of medicine, which provides an insight about the natural history of the disease, i.e. complete course of illness, from its origin to its termination.

Today, we are enjoying the fruits of science, in every field of life, including medicine. Now, sitting in a hospital/dispensary/clinic, we calmly listen to patient's complaints, make diagnosis, prescribe treatment and tell about prognosis of the disease. Just imagine the very first day when a man (physician) examined the/a sick person. How much difficult was that moment? However, man is the most curious creature on this earth. Due to this quality, the progress to present state has taken place. We can say, the very first physician on this earth, with a keen sense of observation and having a question mark in the mind, was an early epidemiologist.

In today's perspective, suppose a physician is sitting in a dispensary and a patient comes with a complaint of fever. Fever is accompanied with chills and rigor; fever

3

comes every alternate day. These signs and symptoms coincide with a disease entity known to him as malaria. Physician makes the diagnosis and gives treatment. After a few days, another case of fever reports to him. But this type of fever is of low grade, continuous and it is also associated with pain in abdomen. Another day a new patient visits the physician with a complaint of fever, cough, loss of appetite, etc. The physician is only aware about malaria or we can say for him fever and malaria are synonymous.

If the physician is a good observant and of curious nature, he will definitely think that the other two types of fever are different from the first one, i.e. malaria.

He will explore in depth. He will ask more questions and will compare the three fevers. A good clinician will make a record and categorize the patients accordingly. He will try to find some links as:

- One type of fever is associated with density of mosquito, present in that area.
- Another type of fever is having relation with intake of contaminated water.
- Third type of fever is having some relation with air pollution or cigarette smoking.

'Asking questions and making comparisons' is the name of science which is dealt by epidemiology or these are two keywords of Epidemiology.

It is a science, which is as old as the story of Adam and Eve, who were not allowed to eat the forbidden fruit and the creative man's mind suddenly argued, 'why?' and the epidemiology came into existence. In fact, who, when, where, what, why are the starting words of epidemiology.

Even today, we come across patients with some unknown, deviant signs and symptoms or some new disease entity like AIDS and Ebola which is not known to medical science. And when they come into picture, they challenge our knowledge. So, epidemiology is a science to explore unusual happenings. Cholera was an unusual happening hundreds of years back and AIDS was a challenge about two decades back and still today, we are confronted with situations we don't have an answer to.

But we have learnt the procedure. We know the epidemiological methodology by which we can find the fruitful inferences about new phenomenon.

It is just like solving a quiz problem.

How to reach the solution of an unknown problem, an unknown disease:

1. To whom it effects : Animal/human/vegetation
2. Male or female : Equally
3. Out of children : Infant, pre natal, post natal, neonatal
4. Congenital or infectious? : Infectious
5. Viral/bacterial/parasitical? : Viral
6. Which system it involve? : Gastrointestinal
7. Related with mother's infection? : No
8. Which is the first symptom? : Diarrhea
9. Related with which event? : Eating outside/while on trip
10. ....

Of course, it is a mind-set to be 'curious'. It is not simply accepting what others have said but to reach a conclusive inference.

The well accepted definition of Epidemiology is the study of frequency, distribution and determinants of health related states or events in a specified **population** and the **application** of this study to the control of problems.

KEYWORDS

Epidemiology in its definition has following keywords:
- Health related states and events
- Human population
- Distribution
- Determinants
- Frequency

Health Related States and Events

As already explained, it's not just the study of epidemic or disease but study of all kinds of defects, disorders, disabilities, injuries, genetic traits, physiological conditions; like pregnancy, lactation, infancy, adolescence, socio-pathological conditions; like drug addiction, educational awareness, knowledge, attitude and practices in various health care facilities, etc. i.e. all situations directly or indirectly related with health.

Human Population

Epidemiology is concerned with both sick and healthy population with 'community' as its laboratory. It studies the whole population, a representative sample of it or in its high risk section, depending upon the objective of the study.

Distribution

This is an area concerned with when, where and whom, i.e. time, place and person distribution of health related events.

a. *Time distribution:* Concerned with behavior of disease over the hours of the day (diurnal distribution), months of the year (seasonal distribution), years of decade (cyclic distribution) and decades of centuries (secular distribution).

b. *Place distribution:* Gives an idea about the geographic distribution of the disease, i.e. which states of the country, which districts of the state and, village and mohalla? Urban and rural are the general expressions in place distribution.

c. *Person distribution:* Presents the magnitude of the disease by age, sex, caste, socio-economic status, literacy, occupation, etc.

Determinants

These are the answers to why? i.e. the factors responsible for the causation of the disease. They study the health related events in terms of agent, host and environment.

Frequency

It refers to the load of disease and magnitude of problem. It is studied as rates and ratio. Specifically, when new cases are to be studied in a particular period, term 'incidence of disease' is applied and for total new and old cases, term 'prevalence' is used.

Application

It is the ultimate step after knowing the distribution and causes of disease. This knowledge is used for planning Health Programmes.

It is a science, as it has various study design which gives the answer to who, what, when, where and why and an art as all those findings are very well applied on the human population to minimize the sufferings (Table 1.1).

Table 1.1: Epidemiology sum up

Disease frequency	Distribution	Determinants

(Rates/Ratio)
– Incidence
– Prevalence
– Morbidity/Mortality
	(When, Where and Who)
	According to
	  – Time
	  – Place
	  – Person
		(Why)
		– Cause or etiology
		– Risk factors
		  • Agent
		  • Host
		  • Environment

Comparison	Patterns of disease among subgroups	Scientifically sound health programme can be started

Clue for etiology
Strategy for control and prevention
Health related events in community
– Needs
– Demands
– Activity
– Tasks
– Health care utilization
Magnitude of problem and then planning
	– Age
	– Sex
	– Caste
	– Religion
	– Socio-economic status
	– Marital status
	
	Planning and Management at administrative level
		Some policies for Long Term Management can be made.
		  • Cessation of cigarette smoking
		  • Age of marriage
		  • Food adulteration act
		  • Population policy

CHARACTERSTIC OF EPIDEMIOLOGIST AND CLINICIAN

EPIDEMIOLOGIST

Unit of study is defined as the population or population at risk for which the investigator goes to a community (field).

Concerns with

- disease pattern in entire population
- both healthy and sick population
- conceptual and social aspects, etc.
- data derived from study
- tables and graphs to draw inference
- relationship between cases/population in the form of rates
- comparison between two groups

Seeks

- to identify a particular source of infection
- mode of spread
- to identify etiological factors
- weighs, balance and contrast about crucial difference in host and environmenta factors

Needs

- definition of disease, which should be precise, valid, acceptable and applicable in large community and enable him to identify a person who is diseased
- **Recommend:** specific control measures
- **Evaluate:** outcome of preventive and therapeutic measures (feedback)
- **Determine:** future trends

CLINICIAN

- **Unit of study** is cases or patients
  - Patients comes to O.P.D (hospital- clinic)
- **Concerns with**
  - Disease in individual patient (period of pathogenesis)
  - Sick persons only
  - Biomedical concepts
  - Advanced techniques of diagnosis and treatment, i.e. clinical examination, lab diagnosis, postmortem
  - Interested in host or at the most agent
- **Seeks**
  - A diagnosis and then prescribe treatment
- **Needs**
  - Not required disease definition–one can make presumptive diagnosis and can revise the diagnosis afterward
  - **Recommend** – treatment
  - **Determine** – prognosis of disease, i.e. DISEASE is the only consideration

Epidemiologists and clinicians are not two opposite ends, but they are mutually helpful to each other. Disease identity is important for an epidemiologist and prevention, etiology and prognosis is important to a clinician.

SCOPE OF EPIDEMIOLOGY

Epidemiology, as defined by 'Last', concerns not only disease and death components but also other health related events. In this way, it also gives indication to improve upon the situation after knowing the distribution and determinants of disease or events. So in this way, epidemiology is a basic medical science with the goal of improving the health of populations.

The scope of epidemiology can be:

1. **Causation of disease:** The knowledge of distribution of disease in terms of time, place and, person provides hypothesis and this is further tested and confirmed by various epidemiological studies. These causative factors may be genetic or environmental or it may be causation of both which leads to ill health.

2. **Natural history of disease:** Epidemiology is a very important and significant tool to study the natural history of any disease. Epidemiologists study the disease pattern in the community in relation to agent, host and environmental factors. One can study a complete pattern of disease starting from good health, subclinical disease, clinical disease, disability and recovery from disease or even death.

3. **Classification of disease:** The epidemiological observations suggest that various diseases are having different determinants and should be classified accordingly, e.g. peptic ulcer group should not include gastric and duodenal ulcer as one, as they are different in etiology. Similarly vehicle and vector borne diseases are classified according to their key determinant. These provide an insight for further management.

4. **Description of health status of population:** Epidemiology is often used to describe the health status of population groups. Knowledge of the disease burden in population is essential for health managers who guide us, in relation to limited resources for the best possible effect.

5. **Evaluation of intervention:** These days epidemiologist are involved in evaluating the effectiveness and efficiency of health services by determining the appropriate length of stay in hospital or community interventions for specific conditions under national health programmes.
   - Treatment regimen for blood pressure in diabetes
   - Efficiency of sanitation measures to control diarrheal diseases.
   - Input of vitamin A supplement, iron and folic acid tablets.
   - Utilization of health services, i.e. knowing about OPD attendance.

USES OF EPIDEMIOLOGY—FLOW CHART

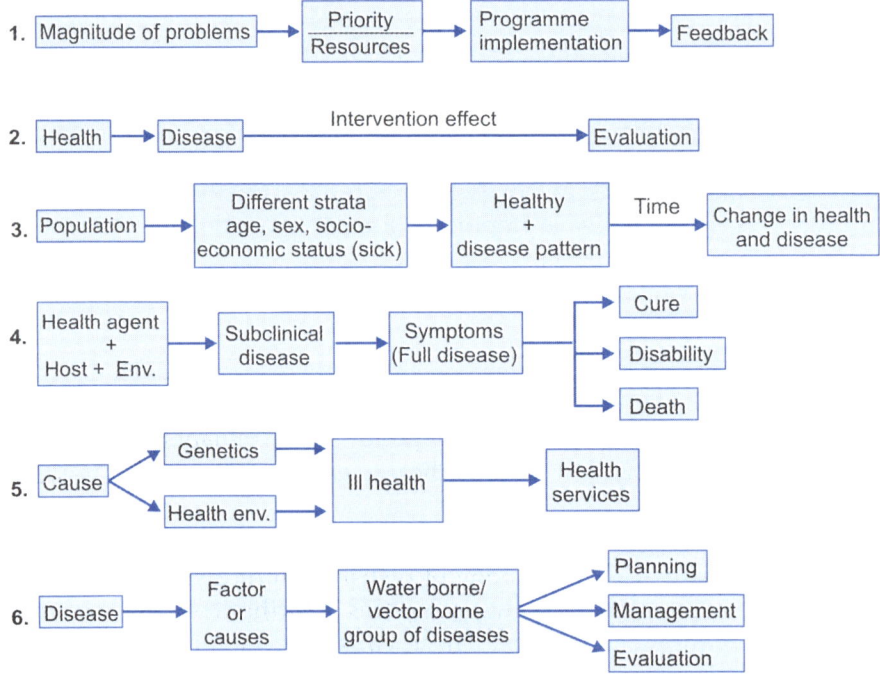

6. Planning: The planning of any community or country is the hallmark of development. Similar is the case with health planning.

- Epidemiology provides indices, which is important to know the load of problems. In its first step, it provides a list of problems.

- Planning starts when the magnitude of problem is in hand. Then these problems are prioritized, keeping in view the resources of the country.

HISTORICAL EVENTS

If we trace back the origin of epidemiology in modern medicine, the following events have their pioneer position:

Hippocrates have mentioned in his book on "air, water and places and also about seasons, winds, rising sun, etc. somewhere about twenty five centuries back. Some physician said that Hippocrates used the word 'consider' not 'count', but definitely Hippocrates have the pioneer place, when today we talk about relationship between man and environment.

John Grant while working on the bills of mortality in London in 1662, made an attempt to give numerical value to the events.

Not only science but the total development of human beings is due to their keen observation in the natural events of their surroundings. It may be the observation of **Newton** about falling an apple on earth or it may be an observation of **John Snow** about disease of cholera, who formulated his hypothesis in the year 1849 before the invention of microscope or even knowledge about microscope, that cholera is related with drinking contaminated water and signs and symptoms are due to lesions in the intestine.

Mr. Lind tried fresh fruits in the treatment of scurvy in 1747.

Jenner's experiment in 1796 with cowpox vaccine is a landmark in the field of immunization.

In 1905 **Fletcher** assessed the protective effect of curd rice against beri-beri in Kuala Lumpur lunatic asylum, which was previously considered a contagious disease.

Goldberger inducted the pellegra by deficient diet in 1915.

STRATEGIES OF EPIDEMIOLOGY

Facts exist in nature. Inquisitive mind examines or observes these facts and wants to correlate and formulate certain conclusions, which in scientific language are known as hypothesis formulation (yet to become a theory). Now he is interested in analyzing these facts. He obtains additional information. He designs some scientific study and further observes to analyze the facts. If necessary, he makes a deliberate intervention in the situation, if possible and wants to know new facts and so on.

Suppose a scientist observes that lung cancer is more common among cigarette smokers, then he plans another study to know more facts, so that his research gets strengthened. He observes its relation with number of cigarette smoked in one day, type of cigarette (filter/nonfilter) a person is smoking, duration of smoking as compared to non-smokers and within smokers. Further he noticed its relation with various chemicals like tar, nicotine and carbon monoxide, etc.

Strategies of Epidemiology

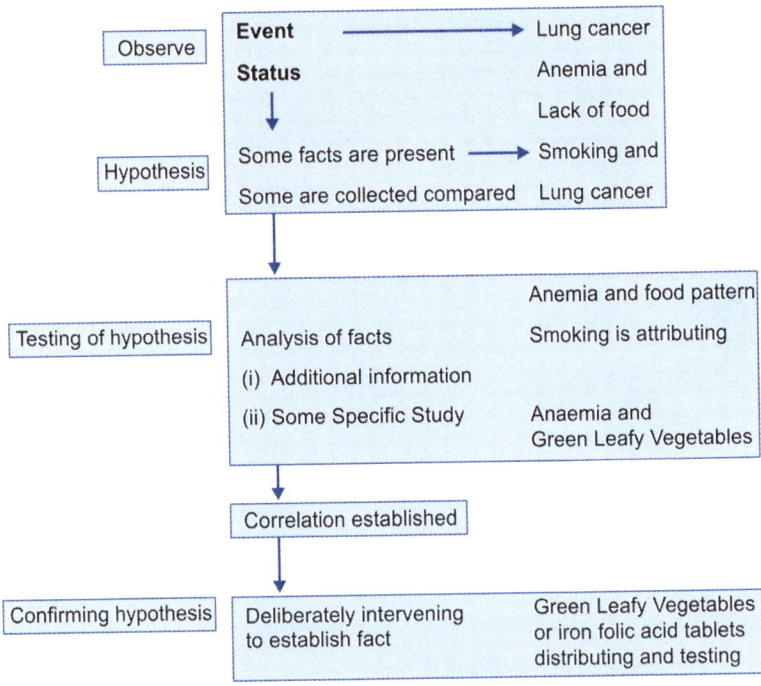

So first he observes and describes, then observes and analyzes and at last, if required he deliberately manipulates and conducts an experiment. This is how a scientist proceeds. These various steps are known as various types of epidemiological study designs or strategies of epidemiology. This will be discussed under the headings of:

- Descriptive Epidemiology
- Analytic Epidemiology
- Interventional Epidemiology

2

Measuring Health and Disease

Health as perceived by anyone in the society gives multifaceted impression. We usually use 'health is wealth'. 'Health is a major social investment', it is an asset and linked with productivity and prosperity.' On the other hand world health organization (WHO) defines health as a state of complete physical, mental and social well-being and not merely the absence of disease or infirmity.

But when coming to measurement of health, it provides more of a conceptual and abstract aspect which is not so easy to measure. We can describe positive and negative indicators of health. Positive indicators of health include mean birth weight, mean life expectancy and mean anthropometric value. Some other indirect indicators are gross national product, adult literacy, access to safe water supply, access to basic sanitation and access to health services.

If we talk of negative indicators of health, then it means we are talking in terms of disease. Similarly disease is a state of departure from health. The word disease itself is made of two words, 'dis + ease' means not at ease or not feeling comfortable. We can simply measure the disease by saying it is present or absent. But it is not that simple when it is to be measured at mass level. Sometimes disease can be said to be present with single sign and symptoms like in 'measles' and in another situation the complex 'syndrome like' picture is present, as in case of AIDS and rheumatic fever.

In clinical practice it is less rigid as the diagnosis of disease can be changed over a period of time, but in epidemiological investigation some definite criteria is required. Whatever decision be taken, it is necessary that disease definition should be clearly stated, easy to use, easy to measure in standard manner under a wide variety of circumstances by different people.

MEASURING THE DISEASE

We can measure the disease from these aspects
- Morbidity
- Mortality
- Disability
- Others

Before going on to the actual measurement, we must be clear about tools of measurements like rate, ratio and proportion, percentage and also about the concept of numerator and denominator.

Rate

It is a measure of frequency with which some event occurs or we can say, it is counting of cases in a defined population. The number of cases alone without reference population (usually population at risk) can occasionally give an impression of the overall magnitude of a health problem or of short term trends in a population, for instance during an epidemic. Rate provides more scientific information and can be used for comparison.

It requires:
- Cases (numerator)
- Population (denominator)
- Multiplier
- Definite area and time period

Ratio

It relates to two random quantities, i.e. numerator and denominator are two different entities. Numerator is not a part of denominator, e.g. male-female ratio in India, RBC to WBC, hip–waist ratio, doctor–population ratio or doctor–nurse ratio, etc.

Proportion

It is a special type of indicator which expresses the relationship between part and the whole. The numerator is a part of the denominator, e.g.

$$\text{Proportional mortality rate} = \frac{\text{Number of deaths due to specific disease}}{\text{Total number of deaths}}$$

for example, one third deaths are due to CVD out of total deaths or one fifth of population is of adolescents.

Percentage

A proportion multiplied by 100 gives the value in percentage, e.g. 20% population of adolescents, 40% population below poverty line.

Numerator

Numerator is the number of cases or number of events, i.e. disease, death, accidents, episodes of disease, i.e. diarrhea, etc.

Denominator

It is the total population of a specific group of people going to be affected by that event or total number of people at risk to that event or disease.

It can be said that the numerator has no value or very little value if the denominator is not there.

To calculate the rate, a relevant denominator is required. Relevant and correct denominator is ideally one, which should include those people, who are potentially susceptible to the diseases/events studied, for example, men should not be included in calculation of the frequency of carcinoma of cervix.

The denominator should be relevant as to highlight the magnitude of problem properly. While calculating birth rate, death rate the whole population (mid-year population which is usually estimated as on 1st July) can be used but otherwise population at risk should be considered, i.e. population which is susceptible to a disease/event, e.g. while calculating general fertility rate, older women and early adolescent girls should be excluded and denominator should be 15–49 years of women.

Some more specific denominator can be used as in case of calculating blindness; the blind hours should be calculated and can be used as a denominator to know the seriousness of the problem.

Similarly for road traffic accidents, number of vehicles or length of roads or other such denominator can be used.

The purpose of denominator is to express the rate in a manner that the frequencies of disease/event being calculated should highlight the true picture of that particular situation.

MEASURING MORBIDITY

Morbidity rates measure the frequency of diseases in a population. Several measures of disease frequency are based on the fundamental concept of prevalence and incidence. It's true that disease severity and disease duration are also measured by case fatality rate and disability rate.

Advantages
i. Magnitude of disease is measured which is further needed for listing the priorities in the community.
ii. Programme planning for prevention and control of diseases.
iii. Monitoring and evaluation of diseases which give feedback for future addition and alteration of strategies.
iv. Prerequisite for basic research.

Difficulty in Measuring Diseases
- Variable course of disease inapparent, subclinical, clinical.
- One person may have many diseases.
- Demographic transition in diseases and their pattern.

Prevalence and incidence are two main epidemiological rates which are most commonly used.

Prevalence and incidence are basically involved in counting the cases in defined population (or population at risk) in a given period.

There are fundamentally different ways of measuring occurrence of diseases and relation between prevalence and incidence varies between diseases.

1. High prevalence low incidence–diabetes, hypertension
2. Low prevalence high incidence–common cold, diarrhea

Diarrhea occurs more commonly than diabetes, but it remains for short a period, on the other hand once diabetes occurs, it is permanent. So time and disease duration is important.

PREVALENCE RATE

It refers to all current cases (old + new) existing at a given point of time or over a period of time in a given population.

$$\text{Point prevalence} = \frac{\text{No. of all persons with the disease or condition at the specified time}}{\text{No. of people in the population at risk at the specified time}}$$

$$\text{Period prevalence} = \frac{\text{Total no. of persons known to have had a disease or attribute during a specified period (say one year, six month etc.)}}{\text{Population at risk of having the disease or attribute midway through the period}}$$

Period prevalence = point prevalence at beginning of specified period + incidence during that period

Period prevalence is of limited usefulness, since both the epidemiologist and administration will generally require knowledge of whether the cases being counted are new or old. So in general when term prevalence is used, it is the point prevalence.
Several factors can influence prevalence rate:

It is increased by
- Longer duration of disease
- Prolongation of life of patients without cure
- Increased in incidence, i.e. if new cases are added more in number
- In migration of cases or susceptible people
- Out-migration of healthy people
- Improved diagnostic facilities, i.e. better reporting of cases

It is decreased by
- High case fatality rate from diseases
- Shorter duration of disease
- Decrease in new cases, i.e. after implementation of programme as in tuberculosis
- Improved cure rate of cases with better and new treatment regimens.
- In-migration of healthy people
- Out-migration of cases (patients)

Uses
1. Prevalence rate are helpful in assessing the need for health care and planning of health services, e.g. hospitals, manpower, etc.
2. Useful for measuring the occurrence of conditions for which the onset of disease may be gradual, i.e. magnitude of health/disease in population. So potentially high risk population is identified.

Limitation
Not ideal for studying disease etiology.

INCIDENCE RATE

Incidence rate is calculation of new cases that develop in a defined period.

It is:

$$I = \text{Incidence rate} = \frac{\text{number of people who get a disease in a specified time}}{\text{Population at risk during that period}}$$

It is important to know that:
- Incidence refers to first event of disease
- It should always include a dimension of time (day, month, year, etc.)
- In disease like diarrhea, acute respiratory infection, malaria, etc. where the duration of disease is small, it can refer to new spells or episodes of disease.
- As the incidence is mostly calculated in many years' time period, i.e. in longitudinal (cohort) studies, then it is better to calculate person-time incidence rate, i.e. each person in the study population contributes one person-year to the denominator for each year of observation before disease develops or the person is lost to follow up.
- If in a population, healthy at the beginning and followed for 5 years, to see the effect of smoking, the population divides naturally into smokers and non-smokers. Suppose the population of an area is 5000, out of which about 1000 person are smokers and 4000 are nonsmokers. Now out of 1000 person, some smoke for two years or so, while calculating incidence rate it should be

$$\frac{\text{No. of new cases developed during the period}}{\text{Total no. of person-year (during these 5 years) of observation}}$$

Importance of Incidence

1. It is a health status indicator, which gives indication for actions to be taken to control disease.
2. Useful indicator for research into etiology and pathogenesis distribution of disease and efficacy of preventive and therapeutic measures.
   If incidence rate is increasing it suggests:
   – Failure or ineffectiveness of the control programme
   – Need for new disease control programme
   – Reporting practices has improved
3. Change or fluctuation in incidence may also mean a change in the etiology of disease, e.g. change in the agent, host and environmental features.

Table 2.1: Difference between incidence and prevalence

Incidence	Prevalence
No. of new cases of a specific disease or no. of Spells/Episode × 100	All current cases (OLD + New) of specific disease at given point of time
Population at risk	Estimated population at same point of time
It is inversely proportional to time $I = \dfrac{P}{D}$	Longer the duration, more is the prevalence, i.e it depends upon time $P = I \times D$
It is a continuous phenomenon as video recording (motion picture)	It is like still photography (just like snapshot)

(Contd...)

Table 2.1: Shows the difference between incidence and prevalence (*Contd.*)

Incidence	Prevalence
It is important in knowing causal factor study between variables	Not ideal for measuring cause
It takes long time, requires period of assessment, i.e. months, years	It is an instant (time saving procedure, easy to measure)
It is usual method of comparison	Comparison is difficult
Useful for epidemiologists, researchers	Administratively useful

MEASUREMENT OF MORTALITY

Uses of Mortality Data

A. Explain trends in mortality pattern

   Priorities for health action

   Designing intervention programme

   Allocation of resources
   ↓
   Assessment and monitoring of public health problems and programme

B. It gives important clues for epidemiological research.

Limitations of mortality data:

1. Incomplete reporting of deaths
2. Lack of accuracy
3. Lack of uniformity
4. Choosing a single cause of death
5. Other diseases and conditions which contribute to patient's death are not tabulated
6. Diseases with low mortality

There is not much of help with mortality data in cases of chronic diseases.

Mortality Rates and Ratios

1. Crude death rate (CDR)

$$= \frac{\text{No. of deaths (from various causes) during the year} \times 1000}{\text{Mid-year population}}$$

Advantage: It portrays an impression of population in a single figure

Disadvantage: Lack of comparability for communication with population that differ by age, sex, race, etc.

Population	CDR	Age specific death rates per 1000 population					
		0–1	1–4	5–7	8–44	45–64	65 +
A	15.2	13.5	0.6	0.4	1.5	10.7	59.7
B	9.9	22.6	2.0	0.5	3.6	18.8	61.7

- Population B appears to be healthier as CDR = 9.9 than population A with CDR=15.2
- In fact population A is healthier as the age specific death rates are lesser as compared to population B
- Higher rate of CDR in population A is due to older population as compared with population B which has relatively younger population.

2. Specific death rate

a. Depending on cause or disease specific.
b. Related to disease group.

Advantages

i. Helps to identify a particular group or groups at risk for preventive action
ii. Permits comparison between different causes within the same population

Disadvantage

Obtained mainly in countries where registration system is perfect and have authentic (Medically Approved) death certificates, e.g.

Specific death rate due to TB

$$= \frac{\text{No. of deaths due to TB during a calender year} \times 1000}{\text{Mid-year population}}$$

3. Case fatality rate (CFR)

a. It is proportion of deaths to cases, so it represents killing power of disease.
b. It is useful only in acute infectious diseases.

$$\text{CFR} = \frac{\text{Total no. of deaths due to a particular disease} \times 1000}{\text{Total no. of cases due to the same disease}}$$

4. Proportional mortality rate

It is the no. of deaths due to a particular cause (or in specific age group) per 1000 total deaths.

Disadvantage

As PMR depends upon 2 variables and not on the total population, so it is of limited value in making comparison with population groups or different time periods.

5. Survival rate

$$= \frac{\text{Total no. of patients alive after 5 years} \times 1000}{\text{Total no. of patients diagnosed with same disease}}$$

Advantages

i. It gives prognosis of certain disease conditions.

ii. If it is taken from start of treatment, this indicator can be used as a yardstick for the assessment of standards.

DISABILITY RATES

Due to intervention of medical technology, death rates are showing static status. In this scenario disability rates related to illness are gaining an important place.

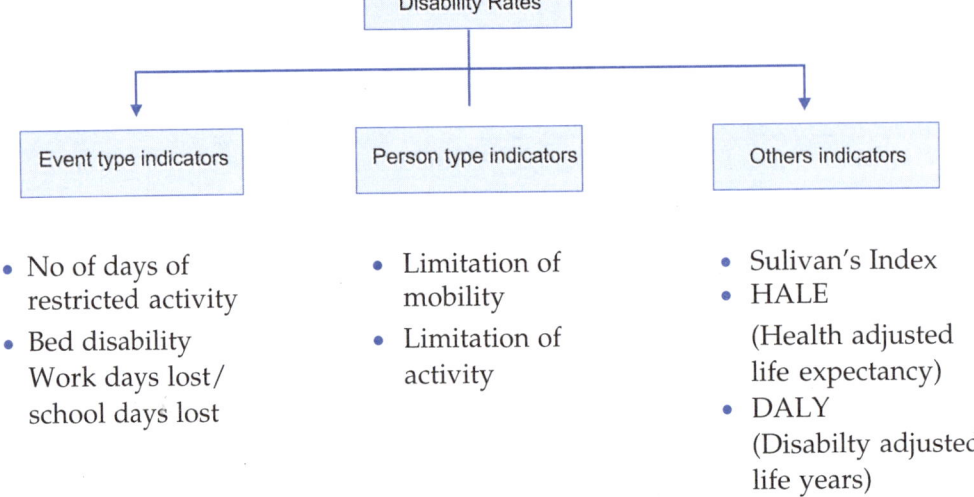

- No of days of restricted activity
- Bed disability Work days lost/ school days lost

- Limitation of mobility
- Limitation of activity

- Sulivan's Index
- HALE
  (Health adjusted life expectancy)
- DALY
  (Disabilty adjusted life years)

Sullivan's Index

It is calculated as:

Life expectancy – (Probable duration of bed disability +
         inability to perform major activities)

Example

L.E = 70 years

Bed disability = 3.3 years

Inability to perform major activities = 1.5 years

Sullivan's index = 70 – (3.3+1.5)

= 65.2 years

HALE (health adjusted life expectancy)

Life expectancy at birth-adjustment for time spent in poor health, i.e. Number of years in full health that a new born can expect to have on current rate of ill health and mortality

DALY (disability adjusted life years)

It is defined as years of life lost to premature death and years lived with disability

1 DALY = one lost year of healthy life

Others: There are other measurements to reflect the health and disease components of society and individual. The important one which are gaining value in these days are nutritional status, socio-economic status, mental health and even health care facilities and environmental status, etc.

Classification of Epidemiological Studies

Epidemiological studies are classified into two major types

- **Observational:** where investigator observes and does not manipulate, the course of disease/event occurs in nature independently.

- **Interventional:** where investigator intervenes/manipulates deliberately. These are also known as experimental studies

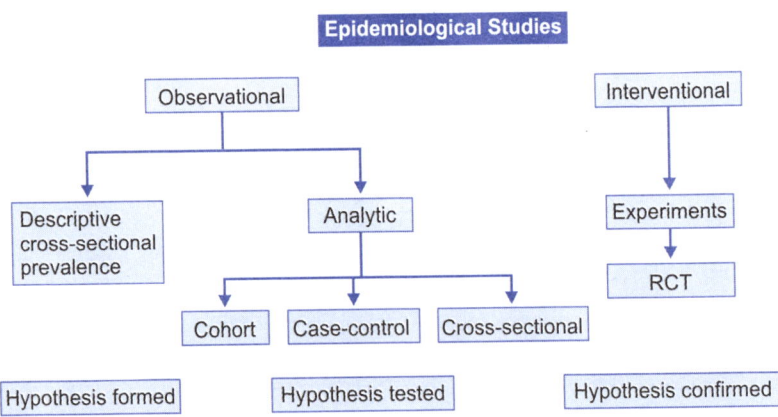

OBSERVATIONAL STUDIES

These are again of two types:

a. Descriptive Studies

They are limited to the description of a disease only and no comparison is made with the reference population.

b. Analytic Studies

They analyze the relationship between health status and other variables like age, sex, socio-economic status, eating pattern, exercise, smoking, etc.

There are various types of analytic studies as
- Ecological and correlational studies
- Cross-sectional studies or prevalence studies
- Case control studies
- Cohort studies

INTERVENTIONAL STUDIES

These are deliberate efforts to change the course of disease. These are of different types as:
- Randomized control trials or clinical trials
- Field trials for healthy population
- Community trials or community interventional studies for communities

DESCRIPTIVE EPIDEMIOLOGY

It studies about distribution of disease.

When ——— Time
Where ——— Place
Who ——— Person

Descriptive epidemiology answers distribution element of epidemiology. It is the first step of an epidemiological investigation. In fact, descriptive epidemiology includes descriptive studies, ecological studies and cross-sectional studies.

Descriptive studies are simple description of health status of a community. Ecological studies are analysis of population or groups rather than individual, on the other hand cross-sectional studies measure the prevalence of the disease and measurement of exposure and effect is also calculated at the same time.

Descriptive studies: These are presented in terms of:
- Disease in community
- Community in disease

DISEASE IN COMMUNITY

It means who are affected, which areas are affected and at what time it shows maximum effect. They basically answer three questions who, when and where or we can say they center around time, place and person.

COMMUNITY IN DISEASE

It means health status of community, i.e. which are the major diseases in the community? Which is the disease of significant severity in terms of disability? Which section of the community are the worst effected?

This type of interpretations about health and disease of community is also known as 'community diagnosis'.

PERSON, PLACE AND TIME VARIATION

Descriptive studies primarily aim at describing the disease or health related events by time, place and person. This is done by collection of data or by already collected data.

One must remember that this is just sorting of data or grouping of variables according to time, place and person characteristics and this must not be interpreted as any association of causal factors.

It can also be understood as the first clue towards the causal relationship which initiates for further queries or further designing of the more detailed studies.

The purpose of categorizing the disease must be kept in mind, i.e. the categorization should be purposeful, so that the inference leads to some scientific designing of next step, i.e. analytic study and fruitful intervention.

PERSON VARIATION

Person can be described in terms of either their inherent or acquired characteristics such as age, sex, race, religion, occupation, marital status, socio-economic status, etc.

These characteristics determine to a large extent that which persons are at greatest risk of acquiring a specific disease.

1. **Age:** It is the most important variable which must be considered in epidemiological studies. For most diseases the variation in frequency that occurs normally due to increasing age are greater than those to be found in association with any other variables. Each infectious disease has its own characteristics age incidence, e.g. measles and whooping cough have their highest incidence between the age group of 1–5 years, while diphtheria and mumps are more common in school going children.

   Association of disease frequency is measured by relating the number of cases in each group to the population in the same group and deriving age specific incidence or prevalence rates.

   Age grouping should be kept relatively small to detect differences. Large groups are likely to hide the age specific incidence in the distribution of cases.

   Age is related with maturity of organ system, efficiency of defense mechanisms and rate of health decline.

   Age indicates the cumulative outcome of a lifelong agent–host interaction. This must be kept in mind that environmental factor is not same in all individual and so is the agent–host interaction.

   Sometimes there may be two separate peaks instead of one in the age incidence curve of diseases as in the case of Hodgkin's disease, leukemia and female breast cancer. It holds special value which indicates that either the data collected is not homogenous or the two different causal factors are operating in the two modes.

2. **Sex:** The study of sexwise distribution of cases and deaths due to a particular disease is a time tested epidemiological practice. Some diseases for obvious anatomical reasons are sex specific. In others an excess of incidence in one sex depends upon more subtle differences in the constitute make up of sexes. But the circumstantial differences are also indicative of the difference in disease incidence.

   Disease like thyrotoxicosis, cholecystitis, diabetes, obesity, arthritis and psychoneurosis are more frequent in women while diseases like peptic ulcer, lung cancer, coronary heart disease and various kinds of accidents are more common in men.

Cultural and behavioral factors also influence the health and disease. Of course the group of diseases related to reproductive health of women especially of pregnancy and childbirth are exclusive to females.

3. **Race/groups/ethnicity/religion/nativity:** The basic point in this is the sharing of same living environment for a long time. They not only share some biological characteristics but also social mechanisms. The grouping of disease according to these groups is more, so it is a stimulus for further studies, that whether the diseases are related to genetic constitution or environmental factors.

4. **Occupation:** The general condition under which a person works (apart from exposure to specific physical and chemical agents) may play an important part in determining his disease experience. For example workers working in the coal mines likely to suffer from silicosis, similarly diabetes and hypertension are more among people, which are working as an executive or have office jobs.

   Occupation also influences the pattern of habits of employees, e.g. sleep, night shifts, tobacco and alcohol consumption and their eating patterns. It is now well evident that workers of call centers are showing new set of diseases.

   Occupation of a person is also used as an index of his socio-economic status and it has its own impact on health and disease.

5. **Marital Status:** When mortality rates among married and unmarried are studied, they show that mortality is less among married. As the married persons feel secure and have a sense of responsibility towards family so they live more. Unmarried people are tense; feel socially unacceptable, so indulge in unhealthy health practices. On the other hand cancer cervix is more among married women. It is almost absent in nuns.

6. **Socio – economic Status:** Socio-economic status is reflection of occupation, education and income of an individual. It, of course, affects the health and disease due to purchasing power of individual, his/her social status in the community and life style due to education and occupation. There is definite and significant difference between various socio-economic groups or different social classes as far as the disease pattern is concerned. It is certain that nutrition, housing, sanitation, stress are various other determinants which are entirely different in all these groups.

7. **Lifestyle:** In present day scenario, a new group of diseases is coming up which has been given the name of lifestyle diseases. It is linked with behavior of human beings. The factors which have proved to be linked with this group of diseases are cigarette smoking, sedentary life style, altered dietary habits, i.e. more inclination towards fast food, ready to eat food, feel good foods and stress.

PLACE VARIATION

Frequency of disease manifestation varies from place to place. A place is considered as a given geographic area. It may be considered in terms of street, ward, city, district, and state, region of a country, entire country and so on. For the purpose of epidemiology, place is also considered in terms of urban or rural, institutional or non-institutional, residential or non-residential, etc.

Factors that govern the distribution of diseases on this planet are extremely varied such as longitude, latitude, attitude, temperature, humidity, rainfall, soil, water, air, plant life, insect life, living habits, food habits, life style, occupation, industrialization and urbanization.

We usually talk about epidemic, endemic and sporadic diseases which describe the disease as cosmopolitan, and is restricted to some areas. But even these are specific terms:

Epidemic: The occurrence of cases in a community or region and illness of similar nature in excess of expectation. The number of cases indicating the presence of an epidemic will vary accordingly to the infectious agent, size and type of population exposed, previous experience or lack of exposure to disease.

Endemic: Constant presence of a disease or infectious agent within a given geographic area.

Pandemic: The occurrence of disease which affects large proportion of the population, occurring over the entire nation, a continent or the world.

The demonstration of an association of a disease with place implies the following:

1. The population in a particular place has the characteristics that in themselves are of etiological importance in the disease and differ from those of the population at other places.
2. Etiological factors are present in the physical, chemical and biological environment of the place.
3. It can be a combination of both.

The distribution of the disease according to place can be studied under the following headings.

a. Global variation
b. Regional variation
c. National variation
d. Urban–rural differences
e. Local variation

a. Global Variation

Table 3.1: Global distribution of diseases

S.No	Area	Disease
1.	South-East Asia, Africa	Tropical disease—Malaria
2.	South and central America	Hot and humid climate—Leprosy
3.	Africa, Latin America, Caribbean	Bancroftian filariasis
4.	South West and South East Asia	Malayan filariasis
5.	Tropical Africa, America	Nectar americanus
6.	South East Asia, India, Japan	Ancylostoma duodenale Carcinoma oral cavity Carcinoma stomach

b. Regional Variation (South-East Asia)

India   Oro-pharyngeal carcinoma

Sri Lanka   Cervical carcinoma

Indonesia   Breast cancer

Magnolia   Stomach cancer

c. National Variation

Table 3.2: National distribution of diseases

Area	Climate	Disease
North-Western state Punjab Rajasthan Uttar pradesh	Hot and dry climate	Trachoma
Sub-Himalayan area		Goiter
South and Eastern Region-Nagaland West Bengal Bihar Tamil Nadu Daman	Hot and humid climate	Leprosy
Northern state		Malaria
Southern state		Filaria

d. Urban–Rural Differences

Table 3.3: Urban–rural distribution of diseases

Urban	Rural
Chronic bronchitis	Skin
Accidents	Zoonotic
Lung cancer	Helminthes
CVD	
Mental illness	
Drug dependence	

e. Local Variation

Clustering of cases may be at global level or country level

– Water borne diseases

– Skin diseases

Importance

- These results stimulate to search for cause–effect relationships between the environmental factors and disease so that preventive measures can be initiated.
- They also provide the regionwise magnitude of the problem within the country.

- Urban–rural differences can reflect the deficiency in medical care, levels of education, sanitation, environmental factors, and social class. This can provide a 'high risk group' for the administrators to work with.
- It is also evident that with the knowledge of agent, host and environment interaction, the scenario of disease in terms of distribution of disease pattern has dramatically changed.

TIME VARIATION

Time is another important aspect, which gives clue in the epidemiological investigation.

We can understand the concept of time according to the length of time necessary for the changes to develop in progression of disease.

It can be studied in following types
- Diurnal variation
- Seasonal variation
- Cyclic or periodic variation
- Secular or long term variation

1. Diurnal Variation

They are the variations shown by a disease within a day, e.g. blood pressure or glaucoma.

2. Seasonal Variation

It is the tendency to high or low incidence shown by many diseases at certain times of the year such as diarrhea in summer season and measles or ARI in winter season. Other vector borne diseases like malaria, dengue, filarial, etc. May and June are known as malaria months. Allergic diseases like hay fever and asthma also show seasonal trends. These are related to the environmental factors, which changes with climate like breeding and feeding habits of disease vectors, housing seasons, indoor and outdoor living pattern of the population.

3. Cyclic Variation

Some diseases show a tendency of periodic recurrence after a fixed period. This trend is related with the herd immunity of a particular area, which decreases to certain level after a fixed period and makes the population prone/vulnerable for that disease.

4. Secular Variation

These changes refer to changes that occur gradually over long periods of time and usually imply changes in disease frequency measured over a period of several years or decades. This trend can be upward or downward as we see in case of diabetes, CVD, obesity, cancers that there is increase in number of cases in last three-four decades. We can also observe that polio, typhoid, tuberculosis and other communicable diseases that are towards decline. This change in either direction can be due to awareness among people and implementation of national health programmes.

Importance

Analysis of cases by time enables the formulation of hypothesis concerning the time and source of infection, mode of transmission and causative agent as well as incubation period. Cases of a particular disease recorded according to date, month, year, etc. also provide definite knowledge about the period of incubation as well as the likely future trend. All these are necessary for planning appropriate preventive and control measures.

EPIDEMIC TRENDS

Apart from these variations, the epidemic trend is also a time trend. Epidemic, as we define today, occurrence in a community or region of cases of an illness or other health related events clearly in excess of normal expectancy.

In occurrence of epidemic, region as well as time are two main points. According to time trends there are following types of epidemics:

1. Point source epidemic
2. Propagated epidemic
3. Mixed type epidemic

Point Source Epidemic

- Exposure to disease agent is brief.
- Simultaneous exposure of all subects
- Cases develop in one incubation period.
- It is explosive clustering of cases with in a small interval of time.
- If we draw an epidemic curve, it will have one peak.
- There is sudden rise and fall also, e.g. after taking measures to improve upon contamination of water, air and food.

Propagated Epidemic

- It is from person to person
- Gradual rise in cases
- Sustained plateau
- Gradual fall
- More likely to occur where large number of susceptible cases are gathered or new susceptible cases arrive regularly
- For example, viral hepatitis, poliomyelitis

Mixed Type Epidemic

- Features of both type
- Starts as explosive and continue
- There is sharp rise, high peak, gradual tail off
- For example, cholera

Intensity of epidemic trend depends upon herd immunity, secondary attack rate and opportunity for contact.

4

Cross-Sectional Studies (Prevalence Studies)

INDRODUCTION

Cross-sectional studies can be categorised as:
- Snap Shot
- Portrait of Community
- Measurement of Exposure
- Effect of Exposure

Cross-sectional studies measure the prevalence of disease and are often called prevalence studies. They are carried out at a single point of time. So they present the snapshot or a portrait of community.

In cross-sectional studies the measurement of exposure and effect are made at the same time, so they are relatively easy.

Design of Cross-sectional Study

Following steps are taken:
1. Defining study population
2. Defining the disease or event
3. Observation and analysis
4. Bias and limitations
5. Advantages and disadvantages

Defining the Study Population

The aim of epidemiology is to know the magnitude of the problem or determinants of disease of the population. The population of course, ideally be whole or total, but most of the time, it is not possible. So in an epidemiological way, sample of the population is taken, which is representative of the population.

On the other hand, the word 'population' is not used in demographic sense, but 'population' is the number of persons required for the study purpose. This may be in hundreds or in lakhs. The population selected can be according to age, sex, occupation, cultural characteristics as per the requirement of study. It can be the whole population of a geographical area or sample from it. The purpose of the study is the first need, which gives the indication of selecting the population. It can be a population at risk, i.e. reproductive age groups of women (15–45 yr), it can be school going children, hospital patients, etc. So it can be a group of people defined in many different ways, i.e. saw worker, labour of construction work.

One more important aspect related to population is that it should be:

- Large enough (sufficient)
- Stable
- True representative–should be part of community and not overtly different.

While selecting the population, specific denominator is finalized as the rates are going to be calculated later and these rates reflect the useful information for future planning.

SAMPLE

It is the selected number of appropriate size of population which enables generalisation/projection of observation over the population from which it is selected.

There are various statistical methods to do sampling. Important ones are simple random sampling, systematic, multistage, multiphase, purposive and cluster sampling.

These methods are discussed in detail in Biostatistics section.

Defining the Disease

The second important aspect in cross-sectional study is the defining disease or condition being investigated. The disease definition has different value for a clinician and an epidemiologist. The clinician can begin with a query for the disease and can proceed for further investigations and observations related to disease development. But for epidemiologist, he is to start with the definition of the disease before he enters into the community for collection of data.

So in this respect, disease definition should be

- accurate
- valid
- applicable to use in population

Now, WHO is providing the standard definitions of various diseases or events or conditions but otherwise, if any criterion is not available or suitable, then operational definition of that condition can be coined.

Once the definition is coined, it should be strictly followed throughout the study. If the investigator proceeds blindly then there can be chances of error and no comparison can be made, which is essential to draw conclusion.

Observation and Analysis

After defining a population and the condition to be studied, the investigator with his/her team visit the field to collect the data (observation). As it is a team work it must be standardized so that the collection of data must be carried out in such a way that they can be directly compared with other observations made by other observers. So in a protocol decide

- which observation is to be made
- choose suitable techniques
- train personnel to use the technique
- test the technique

Choosing techniques, WHO monographs are available, otherwise the techniques going to be adopted should be valid, practical, sufficiently inexpensive, sufficiently precise, e.g. if a simple weighing techniques is to be followed; it should be with minimum cloths (minimal should also be clarified), machine should be accurate and tested before the starting of survey and to be checked time and again against the standard machine.

Training of personnel is very important as there are observer variations. These errors can be

- Between observer variation as in hemoglobin checking
- Within observer variation are that in the beginning the observer is fresh and in good mood and in the evening one can be tired, hurried, irritated due to person's responses, so there can be difference in observations; so all these things are important and should be explained.

The measurement techniques should also be repeatable.

SOME IMPORTANT STEPS FOR FIELD WORK

- Consent of people, co-operation of village chief/head school head or health authorities or factory owner, etc. is essential.
- Clearance from ethical committee, if some procedure, tests or even some information (may be secret) is involved.
- Route of area, its accessibility, maps, etc. if required.
- Timing of survey should also be kept in mind as in villages agricultural activities are to be performed, working hours of people, season should be kept in mind and some religious festivals should also be considered.
- Local area health staff should also be informed and their help should be taken.
- Line of flow should be such that, minimal time should be taken and painful procedures (taking blood or vaginal examination) should be done at the last.
- Field equipment, transport, etc. should be prearranged.
- Ensure co-operation of people to participate.

In any survey, there are always a number of people, who fail to attend for interviews or examination, especially in camp setting. The reason for not attending the camp should be discussed. There may be many reasons as lack of information, unwillingness to participate or any other reason. But, one must remember that those who do not come for interview or participate in survey may be an important group, whose exclusion from the survey will bias the report.

After collection of information the analysis is done, where help of a statistician can be taken. The various methods for analysis are used, i.e.

- Mean and standard deviation
- Prevalence and incidence rate
- Co-efficient of correlation
- Percentages and percentiles

Bias and Limitations

Limitations

It is not easy to assess the reasons for association demonstrated in the study.

The data collected is not much useful for comparison of two situations as there is lack of standardized techniques of interviews. The design of questionnaire and sample should be planned and appropriate to have better comparisons.

Uses/Advantages

- These are relatively easy and economical to conduct.
- Useful for investigating the exposure which is the fixed characteristics of individuals as socioeconomic status, blood groups, etc.
- It is the most convenient first step for investigating the cause during sudden outbreak.
- Data collected in these studies is helpful in assessing the healthcare needs of population.

EXAMPLE OF CROSS-SECTIONAL STUDY

During the year 2002, a survey to know prevalence rate of RTI/STI was carried out. 170 primary sampling units (PSU) were selected at national level, out of which 14 were from Punjab, out of 14, two PSU were from urban and 12 from rural. These PSUs' were surveyed by the staff of medical college of Punjab, 4 each PSUs were to be surveyed by GMC Amritsar and CMC Ludhiana while 3 each were allotted to GMC Patiala and GGS medical college Faridkot (multistage sampling).

Then a training of personnel, who were to carry out the survey, was held at regional level (Punjab, Haryana, himachal Pradesh Chandigarh). Four specialists from each medical college (SPM, obstetrics and gynae, skin and microbiology) received training.

In the study design, 100 people (50 male and 50 female) from 15 to 49 years of age groups by random method were selected. Supposing a PSU (a village) has 600 houses, and then every 6th house was selected and alternatively one male and one female were enlisted for study. If there were two or more members present in a particular house belonging to 15–49 years of age, then one was selected by drawing a lottery. (population).

The criteria for STI/RTI was defined on the basis of clinical examination and laboratory test, which were to be performed by various specialists and a survey performa was to be filled by community medicine persons to know demographic profile and other parameters related to STI/RTI.

The local workers [MPW(M), MPW(F)] and health staff of village along with sarpanch of village was informed to make an arrangement of the survey cum medical camp.

Although it was a survey of specified population, who were provided with a specific color cards, otherwise, it was given a look of general medical camp.

A flow line arrangement was made. There was a general OPD to begin with, then selected (specified population) were to report Community Medicine doctors, for filling Performa. During examination phase, first of all skin specialist carrying out their examination, next was gynecological examination and at the end blood and urine samples were taken.

So, all the steps required for cross sectional study were taken into consideration, i.e. from selection of population, defining the disease and collection of data, i.e. observation at one point of time with a scientific methodology. Flow line arrangement was made so that there should be maximum co-operation and least bias.

Table 4.1: Difference between various observational epidemiological studies

	Characteristic	Cross-section	Case-control	Cohort
1.	Rare disease investigation	No	Yes	No
2.	Rare cause investigation	No	No	Yes
3.	Effect of cause study	Some extent	No	Yes
4.	Multiple exposure study	May be	Yes	To some extent
5.	Time relation	No	No	Yes
6.	Measuring incidence	No	No	Yes
7.	Measuring long latent period	No	Yes	No
8.	Time required	Medium	Medium	Long
9.	Cost involved	Medium	Medium	High
10.	Selection bias	Medium	High	Low
11.	Recall bias	High	High	Low
12.	How to follow up	Not Applicable	Low	High
13.	Confounding bias	Medium	Medium	Low
14.	Power to prove cause	Weak	Moderate	Moderate

CLASSICAL CROSS-SECTIONAL (OBSERVATIONAL) STUDY BY JOHN SNOW

- **Carried out place:** England
- **Problem statement:** Cases of diarrhea (epidemic type).
- **Survey carried out in area:**
  - No. of houses: 66153
  - No. of diarrhea cases: 1361
  - Map prepared for location
- Observations
  1. Clear cut distinction between 2 areas
  2. Further question for cause—water supply
  3. Two companies supplying water—Lambeth and Vauxhall
  4. Analysis was done

Table 4.2: Distribution of death cases due to diarrhea in relation to water supply

Water supply company	No. of houses	Deaths due to diarrhea	Percentage
Lambeth	26107	98	0.37
Vauxhall	40046	1263	3.15

- Result

There were 8.5 times more deaths in case of residents supplied by water from Vauxhall company.

5

Case-Control Studies

DESIGN OF CASE-CONTROL STUDIES

- Observational studies
- Analytic studies (Determinants)
  - Agent
  - Host
  - Environment
- Testing the hypothesis
- Answering the 'why' component of disease/event, i.e. investigating causes of the disease.
- Longitudinal studies (Retrospective)
- Enquiry about the disease or event is in backward direction.

Descriptive epidemiology identifies disease problems and relates the disease to host, agent and environment while analytical and interventional epidemiology confirms or relates the observed association between cause and effect.

Case control studies are the next step in the epidemiological investigation after descriptive studies or cross sectional studies, which provide some clue for making hypothesis. This clue is further investigated to test whether the relationship is significant or not.

Various steps involved are:

- Selection of population or selection of cases
- Defining the disease
- Observation and analysis
- Bias and limitations
- Advantages and disadvantages

Selection of Population

As compared to cross sectional studies, the population in these type of studies is cases and control. Cases are the persons who have suffered from some factor or influenced by a cause. Case is sufferer, where effect has been produced by the factor (cause). The suspected cause, the clue of which has been provided by the cross-sectional studies is kept in mind and cases are taken accordingly and to compare these cases, some control (another group of population) is chosen, in which the effect is not present, so they can be healthy or patient of another disease, but not of the case of that disease, which is under investigation.

So in this study the population under observation is:

- Cases
- Control

Selection of Case

The cases are those in which exposure and disease have already occurred but when study is going to be planned, cases must be defined in terms of disease or eligibility criteria to include the cases in the study. These cases can be from hospitals, i.e. patients visiting for carcinoma lung, may be visiting for hypertension or these cases can be from general population or from the field practice area of community medicine. The number of cases or selection of cases required for a study depends upon the prevalence of disease and sample size can be calculated with the help of statistician (Method of calculating the sample size is discussed in Biostatistics Section).

Selection of Control

This is the most difficult task in the case control studies. Controls, who are disease free individuals, should represent people who would have been designated study cases if they had developed the disease. Control must be as similar to the cases, the disease under study or absence of the exposure of the factor whose influence is been studied. Controls can be selected from the same hospitals but with different disease but important is that these patients must be tested thoroughly to exclude the disease under study. Controls can also be included from same household or neighborhood in a community survey or even though hospital cases can be matched with their neighbor or relatives.

Matching

This is a very important step in case-control study. Matching is prerequisite for comparison between cases and control. Matching is the process of selection of control in such a way that not only they resemble cases (study) in all the attributes that is age, sex, occupation, social status, etc. and free from disease under study but free from the confounding factor.

Confounding factor is one which is associated with exposure and disease, and is distributed unequally in study and control group, i.e. this factor can independently act as a risk factor for the disease development, for example, we know that ageing is related with so many diseases. It acts as an independent factor as for atherosclerosis, development of various cancers, etc. is a concern as far as age association is there. So when we are observing the effect of some other factor as oral contraceptive for carcinoma breast, so while matching the age of both groups should be given a special significance. Similarly relating the food habits with atherosclerosis, the young age group should not be compared/ matched with older ones.

Matching can be done by:

- One to one method: One to one or paired matching is done in twin studies, in which case and control are very closely matched.

- Group matching: Group matching is selecting similar type of control, keeping in view age, sex, social status, etc.

DEFINING THE DISEASE

Disease as already discussed in descriptive/cross-sectional study, the diagnostic criteria must be specified before the study is taken. As in a study carried out regarding risk factors among C.V.D patients, the criteria for cases was on ECG changes and disease was classified:

Class I: Q-wave changes

Complete heart block

Complete left bundle branch block

Class II: H/o myocardial infarction

Frankly inverted T-waves

ST depression of 1 mm or more

Like this we can even adopt the disease criteria from WHO monographs or IDSP modules or we can form our own criteria. But once the criterion is established, it should not be altered throughout the study period.

There should also be eligibility criteria or it can be named as exclusion or inclusion criteria, which should also be determined beforehand.

As in the above case, for inclusion criteria, e.g. the case has to be-new, reporting for the first time, not old one.

Similarly, some exclusion criteria like a particular age group or person from specific geographic area will be excluded, keeping in view the hypothesis of the study.

OBSERVATION AND ANALYSIS

The observation includes collection of data. The purpose of collection of data is to get information about exposure factor. It should be obtained from total population, i.e. cases and control.

It can be obtained by interview, records available with cases or hospital records.

For interview, a structured questionnaire can be prepared, keeping in view all the attributes known to influence the disease.

Measurement is done in the following directions:

- How many cases and control were exposed to the suspected factor, i.e. in the above cited study, i.e. how many of CVD patients were having more total serum cholesterol or having more body mass index.

- Was there any relation with type of personality or it was related to socio-economic status or any other relevant factor.

Table 5.1: Two by two table to establish the relation between cases (disease) and factor (cause)

Suspected factor	Cases	Control
Present	a	b
Absent	c	d
Total	a + c	b + d

In such cases, where these types of attributes are involved, also must be defined earlier that how much BMI is normal and what are the levels of total serum cholesterol. These can be graded or quantified. In the above study as total serum cholesterol < 220 was given '0', 220–260 and more than 260 was given 1 and 2 grades respectively.

Analysis

There are main two inferences, which are drawn from the data
I. To know the association/relationship between factor and disease
II. To know the strength of association
   To know the association, we calculate the 'exposure rate' and to know the strength of association 'risk rate' is calculated.
   The data calculated is compiled in a 2 × 2 (Table 5.1).

EXPOSURE RATE

With this data we calculate exposure rate as:
Exposure rate among
i. Case = $a/a + c \times 100$
ii. Control = $b/b + d \times 100$
   In CVD patients, type A personality and disease, the following is the data in a particular study.
Exposure rate among
i. Cases: $33/35 \times 100 = 94.2\%$
ii. Control: $55/82 \times 100 = 66\%$
   So, we can observe that CVD is more among patients with type A personality as compared to other types of personality (Table 5.2).

Table 5.2: Distribution of cases and control in relation to type of personality

	Cases	Control
Type A personality	33	55
Other	2	27
Total	35	82

RISK RATE: (STRENGTH OF ASSOCIATION)

This is calculated as:
   Risk rate = incidence among exposed/incidence among non-exposed (Table 5.3)

Table 5.3: Distribution of cases and control in relation to total serum cholesterol

Level	Total serum cholesterol	Disease present	Disease absent
0	< 220	132	211
1	220–260	138	81
2	> 260	24	2

   As we know that in case control study, incidence cannot be calculated, because there is no proper denominator or we can say, exact number of population at risk is not known so in this case, to know the strength of association, we calculate odd's ratio.

ODD'S RATIO (OR)

It is ratio of exposure among cases and control.

OR = chance of exposure among cases/chance of exposure among control

$$\text{ODDs' ratio} = \frac{(\text{factor present and disease present}) \times (\text{factor absent and disease absent})}{(\text{factor present and disease absent}) \times (\text{factor absent and disease present})}$$

$$\text{OR} = \frac{a \times d}{b \times c}$$

It is also known as cross-product ratio. As it is not real, it is also known as 'psuedo relative risk'.

In the study of CVD cases the following data was obtained.

CVD patient and level of total serum cholesterol

Comparing (calculating zero level and one level)

$$\text{OR} = 138 \times 211/132 \times 81 = 2.7$$

Calculating zero level and two level

$$\text{OR} = 211 \times 24 /132 \times 2 = 19.18$$

So, it is evident that if the total serum cholesterol level is increased to 1st level as compared to normal (zero level) the risk increase 2.7 fold and if it increases to 2nd level (> 260), the risk increases 19.18 times.

Test of Significance: (refer to Biostatistics–Section II)

There are so many tests available in biostatistics and according to the acquired data these are applied.

Here in this case 'chi- square test' is applied to ascertain whether the relation between total serum cholesterol and CVD is significant or not. For this, 'P value' is calculated, which tells us whether the probability of association between the disease and suspected factor has occurred by chance or by real fact. If the P-value is 0.05 or less than that, the relation is considered significant. The lesser the P-value higher is the significance.

BIAS AND LIMITATIONS

There are following bias observed in case-control study
a. Selection bias
b. Memory bias/recall bias
c. Interviewer bias
d. Confounding bias
e. Berkesonian bias
f. Unacceptability bias

a. Selection Bias

It is bound to occur in case control studies as the cause-effect phenomenon has already occurred. If response rates are different, even then selection bias can occour.

It can be reduced by the method that cases and controls should be drawn from different population, but after proper matching.

Multiple controls should be drawn from variety of sources.

b. Memory/recall Bias

There are two reasons for this bias:

Cases and control have different types of reporting due to their exposure, which has resulted in illness in one and none in other.

There may be faulty memories of an individual.

c. Interviewer Bias

In this case, the interviewer knows who the case is and who the control is. So the approach towards the case is different and towards control it can be casual. A more detailed history is sorted from cases while controls are not devoted so much time. This can be reduced by preparing the series of queries and questions and asking all relevant questions to either group or the interviewer should not be disclosed about the status of cases and control.

d. Confounding Bias

It has already been discussed that how confounding produces the bias. Confounding means a factor which provides misleading estimates of effect.

It can be removed by proper matching.

e. Berkesonian Bias

It is a special type of bias observed by Dr. Berkesonian. It is a selection bias as the control and cases are taken from hospital and there is different rate of admission to hospital for different people with different diseases.

f. Unacceptability Bias

People may not give correct information about their personnel, sensitive issues like sexual practices, drugs, etc. This can be reduced by formulating a questionnaire which is of indirect nature.

ADVANTAGES AND DISADVANTAGES

Advantages

1. Easy to carry.
2. Suitable for rare diseases.
3. Lesser subjects (people) are required.
4. Several risk factors can be studied as many causes of CVD.
5. No issues with of diagnostic criteria, administrative setup, as follow up is not required.
6. No attrition problems.

Disadvantages

1. Incidence rate cannot be measured.
2. Selection of control group is difficult.
3. Attributable risk cannot be calculated, so prophylaxis evaluation is not possible.
4. Recall bias is a main problem.
5. Not suited for evaluation of therapy or prophylaxis of disease.

6

Cohort Study

DESIGN OF COHORT STUDY

- Observational study
- Analytic study
- Testing the hypothesis
- Answering the 'why' component of disease/event
- Forward looking or inquire about disease or event in forward direction so called follow up or incidence studies.
- Starting point is healthy population.

In fact, after cross section studies, or forming a hypothesis, cohort studies should be planned, but due to some limitation, these are not taken. Otherwise scientifically, cohort studies provide best information about causation of disease and most direct measurements of the risk of developing disease.

Cohort study is named so because it is done on cohorts.

A cohort is a group of persons possessing common characteristics. Literally means born together, so it comprises birth cohort, similarly factory workers of same exposure are exposure cohort.

Various steps involved are

- Selection of population
- Defining the disease
- Observation and analysis
- Bias and limitations
- Advantages and disadvantages

SELECTION OF A POPULATION

There are two groups; both are healthy to begin with
1. Study cohort (exposure cohort)
2. Control cohort

As cohort means, sharing common characteristics like age, sex, occupation, income, literary status, marital status, housing conditions, nutritional or food habits, etc. Both groups only differ in suspected etiological factor. Study group is exposed to a factor whereas the control group is not, and after a particular period of time, comparison is made about the outcome of the factor.

According to need of hypothesis, population is selected, as in the Doll and Hill study about 5,9,600 British doctors listed from medical registration of UK.

This enables them to form two cohorts-smokers and nonsmokers, i.e. study group or exposure group; exposed to smoking and non-smoker as control group.

4,0,701 of physicians similar in all aspects like age, education and social class were included in the study.

DEFINING THE DISEASE OR ATTRIBUTE CRITERIA

As we have already discussed in case-ontrol study also, the development of disease or any other outcome must be laid down before starting the study. Even the criteria for social class and other such attributes should be defined and should be strictly followed throughout the study. As smoking is going to cause bronchitis, bronchiectasis or lung cancer, etc. So every condition should be defined beforehand.

OBSERVATION AND ANALYSIS

This is again as in an observational study. As in case of Doll and Hill study, to observe the effect of smoking, study was carried out (period of observation) for 4 years and 5 months. The observation was about death due to lung cancer mainly. The death confirmation was obtained from Registrar General, The General Medical Council and British Medical Association. In this study it was observed that death rate among various categories of smokers (one lakh per year) was as follows:

      Heavy smokers : 224 (*a*)

       Non-smokers : 10 (*b*)

Observation in cohort study depends upon the hypothesis, that it is at regular intervals or at the end of the study or some other protocol is adopted.

Analysis

It is done on two dimensions
1. Exposure rate
2. Strength of association
    It is calculated by:
    a. Relative risk
    b. Attributable risk
    c. Population attributable risk

1. Exposure Rate

It is calculated after compiling the data into 2 × 2 table

Groups	Disease		
	Yes	*No*	*Total*
Study cohort (Exposure +)	*a*	*b*	*a + b*
Control cohort (Exposure −)	*c*	*d*	*c + d*
Total	*a + c*	*b + d*	*a + b + c + d*

Exposure rate (incidence) among

study cohort = $a/a + b \times 1000$

control cohort = $c/c + d \times 1000$

If incidence among study cohort is more than control cohort, it shows the association between disease and suspected factor.

2. Strength of Association

a. Relative Risk

$$RR = \frac{\text{incidence of disease or death among exposed}}{\text{incidence of disease or death among non-exposed}}$$

$$= a/a + b/c/c + d$$

As the name relative risk denotes itself that exposed group is relatively at risk as compared to non-exposed or we can say if protective factor is studied (nutritional factor) the same can be interpreted other way.

Suppose in case of lung cancer and smoking, the answer is 4, then it interprets that smokers are 4 times more at risk for developing lung cancer as compared to non-smoker or those who eat green leafy vegetables (GLV) are at less risk of developing anaemia.

b. Attributable Risk

$$AR = \frac{\text{incidence of disease/event among exposed} - \text{incidence of disease/event among non-exposed}}{\text{incidence of disease/event among non-exposed}} \times 100$$

$$AR = \frac{\dfrac{a}{a+b} - \dfrac{b}{c+d}}{a/a+b} \times 100$$

Here again, as the word attributable means how much risk can be attributed to a particular factor in causation of disease or other way, we can say if this particular factor is removed then the disease incidence can be lowered to this much extent. So it quantifies the avoidable incidence of disease.

Suppose in this case, when lung cancer and smoking habits are compared, the attributable risk is calculated to be 87%, we interpret that 87% risk can be attributable to smoking habit or if we stop the smoking or ban the smoking in the region, the incidence of lung cancer can be lowered by 87%.

c. Population Attributable Risk

PAR = incidence of disease occurring in total population of both groups irrespective of risk factor MINUS incidence of the disease among non-exposed group.

$$= a + c/a + b + c + d - c/c + d \times 100$$

This indicates the avoidable incidence of disease due to exposure in the entire population (both groups).

BIAS AND LIMITATIONS

In cohort study bias can be of the following types:

1. Selection bias
2. Attrition bias
3. Confounding bias
4. Non-response bias
5. Measurement bias

Selection Bias or Attrition Bias

As usual, the selection of healthy and comparable cohort (study and control) is difficult to have all the attributes similar.

The subjects (participants) have to be followed for a long period, so it is difficult to have contact. There is always decrease in number due to death or migration or any other reason. This is also termed follow up bias.

Confounding Bias

If the confounding factor is distributed unequally between two cohorts (exposed and non-exposed) the results can be distorted.

Non-Response Bias

There is always a factor of non-response among the participants included without their will, so there is poor response if the number of such participants varied into two groups, it leads to bias.

ADVANTAGES AND DISADVANTAGES

Advantages

1. Incidence rate can be calculated.
2. Dose-response ratio can be measured.
3. Estimation of relative and attributable risk can be done, so prophylaxis programme and strength of association can be predicted.
4. Several outcomes related to exposure can be studied simultaneously. As in case of evaluating the outcome of smoking; apart from lung cancer, CHD, peptic ulcer, bronchitis, etc. can be studied.
5. Certain form of bias can be minimized.
6. Better study design.

Disadvantages

1. Unsuitable for investigating uncommon diseases.
2. Take long time to complete study and obtain result.
3. Administrative problems.
4. Expensive.
5. Ethical problems.

Table 6.1: Difference between case-control and cohort studies

S.No	Case-control study	Cohort study
1.	Effect to cause	Cause to effect
2.	Diseased cases	Healthy persons to start
3.	Few suspect/cases	Large subjects/cases
4.	Incidence rates cannot be calculated	Possible to calculate incidence rate
5.	Odds ratio is calculated to know the strength of association (pseudo relative risk)	Relative risk and attributable risk is calculated
6.	Short duration	Long duration

(Contd.)

Tabel 6.1: Difference between case-control and cohort studies (*Contd.*)

S.No	Case-control study	Cohort study
7.	Quick results	Long follow up
8.	For rare diseases	Inappropriate
9.	Economical	Expensive
10.	More bias	Less bias
11.	More than one factor can be studied	More than one outcome is studied
12.	First approach towards test hypothesis	Reserve technique for next-step
13.	Fairly good study design	Best study design for causal association

Tabel 6.2: Difference between relative and attributable risks

S.No	Relative risk	Attributable risk
1.	Assess etiological role of factor	Assess the contribution of etiological factor
2.	Depict strength of association between cause and effect	Reflect public health importance
3.	Tell about impact of successful public health programme	

CLASSICAL COHORT STUDY: THE FRAMINGHAM HEART STUDY

Problem statement: to study the relationship of a no. of factors to the subsequent development of CVD.

Variables: Serum cholesterol, blood pressure, weight and smoking

Selection of cases (cohort):

Total population of town: 2,8,000 in 1948

Age group selected: 30–59 yr

Person from both sex invited: 6,507

Participated (reported): 5209

Exclusion criteria: already suffering from CVD–82

Actual participants (30–59 years person after all matching): 5,127

Follow up person: 20 years

Subsequent examination: 2 years

Analysis of 1 variable is given in Table 6.3:

Table 6.3: Six year incidence of CHD in relation to serum cholesterol in men aged 40–59

Serum cholesterol (mg/100 ml)	Number	Cases	Rate	Incidence	AR	RR
<210	454	16	0.035	0.0059	0	1.00
210–244	455	29	0.063	0.0106	0.028	1.81
>245	422	51	0.12	0.020	0.085	3.39

Results

Persons with serum cholesterol level >245 are at more than 3 times higher risk for developing CHD.

7

Experimental Epidemiology (Interventional Studies)

INTRODUCTION

Descriptive epidemiology is a cross-sectional study, analytic epidemiology is an observational study while **Experimental epidemiology** is interventional study.

Descriptive epidemiology helps to formulate hypothesis, in analytic epidemiology, hypothesis is tested while in **Experimental epidemiology** hypothesis is confirmed.

Descriptive and analytical studies are about asking questions and making comparisons (simply observing) while **Experimental epidemiology** in addition includes deliberate intervention.

In descriptive epidemiology, we try to see the relationship between agent, host and environment, i.e. association of various variants. Analytical epidemiology measures the strength of association and Experimental epidemiology gives us the information about causal relationship between variants.

Experimental studies involve some action, intervention or manipulation in the experimental group, while making no change in the control group and observing the outcome of experiment (intervention or manipulation) and comparing both the groups.

In fact, man has learnt this technique from nature. Epidemic of cholera, studied by **John Snow**, divided the population into two groups without their own choice. The experiment was done by nature, which is not possible deliberately in all the conditions. But whenever, it is possible, scientists have followed the same aspect knowingly, e.g. **James Lind** performed an experiment and proved that soldiers who were given oranges and lemons for six days recovered from scurvy.

Goldberg's clinical experiment proved pellagra to be a nutritional deficiency disease and not a skin infection as was then supposed.

In present day scenario, in experimental studies, ethical consideration is very important as no patient should be denied appropriate treatment as a result of participation in an experiment and treatment to be tested should be in light of the current knowledge

These are the following types of experimental studies:

1. Randomized controlled trials
2. Field trials
3. Community trials

RANDOMIZED CONTROLLED TRIALS (RCTs)

The study design is having following steps:

1. Selection of population
2. Defining the disease/event or outcome
3. Observation, intervention and analysis
4. Bias and limitations
5. Advantages and disadvantages

1. Selection of Population

a. **Reference population:** It is the population to which the findings of the trial are applicable. This population can be a whole country, even whole mankind, region, village, factory workers, school children or reproductive age group between 15 to 45 years. Also known as reference population.

b. **Sample:** It is not possible to include or carry out a study among reference population (may be a specific group). So a sample is drawn from the reference population. It is the population, the results of which are going to be implemented. So a great precaution needs to be taken to select a sample representative of the reference population, i.e. similarity in demographic characteristic should be there. Incidence of disease to be presented should correspond in both populations.

Population should be suitable practically, i.e. accessible, co-operate, not migratory

The sample size should be according to the statistical technique.

The minimal sample size, i.e.

In qualitative analysis—SEP = $\dfrac{\sqrt{p \times q}}{n}$

In quantitative analysis—SEM = $SD/\sqrt{n}$

(where n = size of sample, SD = standard deviation, SEP and SEM = standard error of proportion and mean respectively)

According to the need of hypothesis or problem statement, the sampling technique should be adopted, which is necessary to minimize the bias.

The various sampling procedures are the subject matter of statistics.

The purpose of the whole exercise is that the reference population (whole) and experimental population (in which study is to be taken) should not be different.

Potential participants

After calculating the sample size and applying sampling procedures the selection criteria is applied to this population. As, who is to be included in the experiment. As in case of diabetes mellitus drug trial, say all new cases will be included or in case of interventional study of anemia, the women having less than 10 gm hemoglobin will be included or there can be exclusion criteria, i.e. the women already taking folic acid tablets or pregnant women or the women of age more than 50 will not be included. So all this should be decided first.

So in this way after applying exclusion and inclusion criteria potential participants are invited for the experiment.

Flow chart of RCT study design

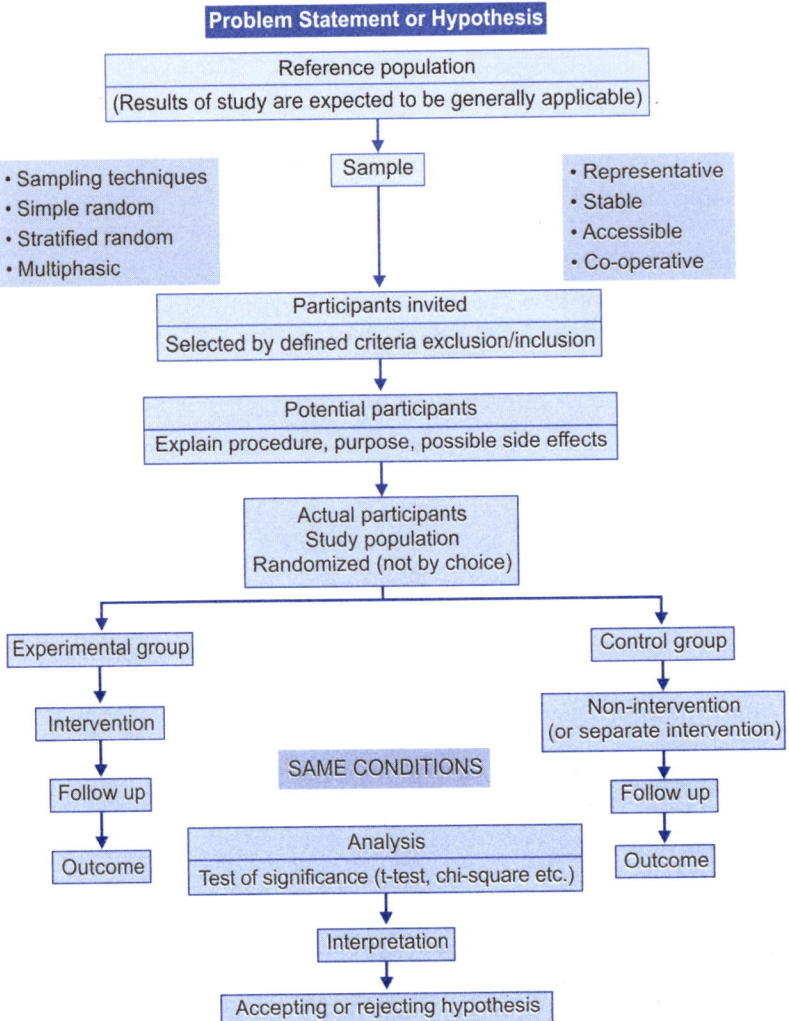

Experimental group

The potential participants, after selection, are explained the purpose of the experiment and the procedure which is going to be carried out. The time, the investigation, the intervention, i.e. the total protocol is explained to them. They are also made aware about the possible side effects of the experiment. In this way, their consent is taken, i.e. whether they are willing to participate or not or they will be available for study period and at time to time for follow up.

Now those who agreed to it are the actual number of persons who are going to be part of experiment. So, keeping in view all the steps, the number of participants should be more in the beginning as calculated by sampling size, otherwise also, the more the size of sample, reliable are the results.

The last step in the selection of population is that the experimental group is divided into two groups randomly (not by choice) into study group, in which intervention is going to apply and control group where no intervention will be there.

So in a nutshell, study group and control group are two parts of selected, potential participants which are sample from reference population.

2. Defining the Disease Event or Outcome

The protocol of the experiment is defined beforehand. All the attributes, variable and disease entity or any type of outcome should be defined clearly so that the end result may be interpreted correctly without any bias. It may be classification of social class, literacy status, grades of malnutrition, level of hypertension, etc. In case of disease entity, for example, level of Hb for anemia and the methodology to measure anemia should be selected before starting the study and it should be same throughout the study.

WHO criteria or IDSP guidelines can be followed for all these types of conditions wherever these are available.

3. Observation, Intervention and Analysis

After selecting the study and experimental population, the important step is randomization. Randomization is a statistical procedure by which the actual participants are allocated into study and control groups. It is necessary for comparison. Randomization means that investigator has no control over allocation of either group, otherwise it can lead to bias. This random distribution can be a simple one where the list is procured and alternate number is allotted to either group or it can be stratified first according to variables and subgroups and the subgroups are randomly distributed into two groups.

Randomization is followed by intervention or manipulation. The intervention can be a deliberate action of applying or withdrawing or reduction of suspected causal factors as per requirement of hypothesis.

So here intervention acts as an independent variable whose effect is then measured.

As per the requirement of the interventional study to see/note the effect of manipulation, some time period is required. So according to the need of the study, a follow up period is there.

If regular examination is required or final outcome is to study, it must follow few basic requirements:

- It should follow standard procedure
- It should be of equal intensity as was prior to the experiment (at start)
- Every individual be followed under same given circumstances
- The framework should be kept same till the final assessment of outcome
- Interval of follow-up should also be definite

Analysis of outcome or regular follow-up, at the end of study should be done by calculation of probability (P-value) or correlation or regression coefficient keeping in view the type of data, i.e. whether it is qualitative or quantitative data, then results should be drawn.

4. Bias and Limitation

i. *Selection bias*

Patient's included in clinical trials are inherently biased due to their stage of illness, so inclusive and exclusive criteria should be stringently followed.

Selection bias is also seen when only volunteers are used, which limits the representativeness.

ii. *Observational bias*

It can be of subject variation and investigator variation

If subject knows he/she is using a new drug, there can be a psychological feeling of wellbeing and similarly, if the investigator knows about drugs/ intervention given to two different groups then unconsciously there can be uneven reporting.

iii. *Placebo effect bias*

In most trials, one group (study) is given the actual drug and other group (control) is given simulated kind of capsules or tablets having some sweetener. As the control group does not know that they are getting only placebo, so they may also report some beneficial effect unconsciously.

These errors can be reduced by

- using strict inclusion/exclusion criteria
- proper randomization
- concealing the identity of intervention from subjects, observers and analysts by single blind, double blind or triple blind methodology.

These types of methodologies are given in Table 7.1

Table 7.1: Various types of blinding methods

Type	Volunteer (subject)	Investigator (observer)	Statistician (analyst)
open	+	+	+
single blind	–	+	+
double blind	–	–	+
triple blind	–	–	–

In open study, everybody knows what is given in trial. In single blind study, subjects are unaware of intervention, while in double blind subjects and observer, both do not know about the manipulation. In triple blind, there is codification from the beginning and the results are decoded after statistical work is over. Mostly double blind studies are done in clinical trials.

ADVANTAGES AND DISADVANTAGES

Advantage

They technically resemble laboratory experiments, so give better understanding of cause–effect relationship.

Disadvantages

- Compliance gets compromised when participants fail to cooperate.
- Ethical question is also important as safety and welfare of participants is related to it, so all procedures are not possible.

EXAMPLE OF INTERVENTIONAL STUDY OF VICTORIA (AUSTRALIA)-1971

Problem statement: Effect of adoption of compulsory seat belt in Victoria–1971 compared with others states where similar legislation was not introduced.

Total participants: 12,918

1. Experimental group: Victoria population with seatbelt: other states without such intervention
2. Follow up: 1 year
3. Outcome: injuries and deaths

Analysis of Data

Table 7.2: Distribution of deaths, injuries, and cases in relation to use of seat belts

	Victoria		Other states	
	Deaths	*Injuries*	*Deaths*	*Injuries*
1970	564	14620	1426	39980
1971	464	12454	1429	40396
%	–17.7	–14.8	0.2	1.0

Results

This is not a randomised control trial, but one can percieve the essence of interventional studies.

Difference is statistically highly significant, i.e. effect of seat belt in prevention of death and injuries is present significantly and further it can be used as a strategy for prevention of road traffic deaths and injuries.

8

Screening for Disease

DEFINITION

Apart from diagnosed cases, the other types of disease category cases are manifold, which in epidemiological term are expressed as submerged cases or phenomenon of 'iceberg'.

These disease cases may be in the form of subclinical cases, carriers, undiagnosed cases. These cases are apparently healthy and therefore not recognized and constitute a mass of unrecognized cases of disease in the community and are responsible for the constant prevalence of the diseases and these hidden cases are a challenge for control and prevention of diseases.

Screening is defined as the search for unrecognized disease or detect for test, examination or any other procedures in apparently healthy individual.

The objective of the screening is to provide treatment to those detected persons either to

• break the chain of transmission or
• prevent the person from long term complications of the disease

USES OF SCREENING

1. Detection of cases and their treatment
2. To prepare strategy to control diseases in community
3. To educate people about advantages of early detection
4. Research purpose

The definite difference between screening and diagnostic tests are given in Table 8.1.

Briefly these can be tabulated as

Table 8.1: Difference between screening and diagnostic tests

Scope	Screening test	Diagnostic test
Subject	Apparently healthy people	Sick people
Approach	Done on group	Individual
Investigation/Researcher	Epidemiologist	Case
Outcome	Test results are final	Indicative

(Contd.)

Table 8.1: Difference between screening and diagnostic tests (*Contd.*)

Scope	Screening test	Diagnostic test
Purpose	To establish community diagnosis	Not final but correlated with condition of the patient
Usefulness	To start control programme	Diagnosis of the patient
Initiation	Education/Planning	To treat the patient
Expenditure	Less	More

Flow Chart of Screening Tests

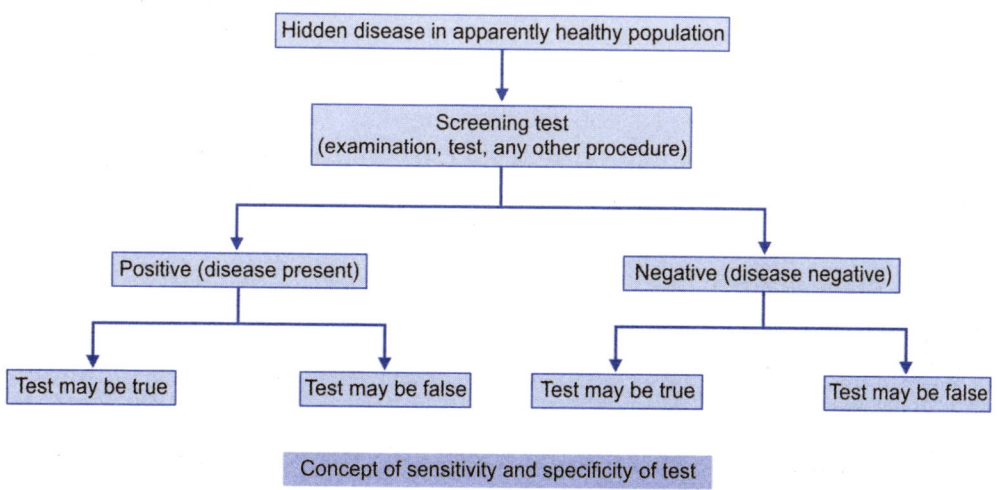

Concept of sensitivity and specificity of test

TYPES OF SCREENING

There are mainly four types of screening procedures
1. Mass screening
2. High risk screening
3. Multipurpose screening
4. Multiphasic screening

Mass Screening is for entire population of an area. However, this is not a useful preventive measure unless it is backed up by treatment and follow-up.

High risk Screening is for those groups of population, who are at high risk of the disease/problem/condition. Cases of high risk pregnancies, women of low socio-economic status for carcinoma cervix or obese persons for hypertension, etc.

Multipurpose Screening is for a group of population by using two or more tests at one time as in case of *antenatal care* groups women when Hb, VDRL, blood grouping, Rh typing and HIV testing is done.

There is one more method, i.e. screening of patients who comes to clinic for other purpose or student entering into college, i.e. opportunistic screening.

Multiphasic Screening is done in various phases as in diabetes, first phase is urine testing and if urine is positive for glucose then second phase is for Fasting Blood Sugar.

Characteristics of Diseases to be Screened

- Should be a public health problem
- Recognizable at early stage
- Should have a test by which the disease can be diagnosed before the onset of signs and symptoms
- Facilities should be available to confirm diagnosis
- Must have effective treatment
- Should have good prognosis with treatment

Criteria for Screening Test

- Should be simple, specific
- Economical
- Rapidly applied
- Acceptable by the people, i.e. not embarrassing
- Reliable, i.e. repeatable and reproducible (should have same result in same conditions, if repeated)
- Valid, i.e. accurate

Variations of the test can be due to:

- Observer
- Biological changes
- Mechanical

CALCULATION AND INTERPRETATION OF SCREENING TESTS

It can be well understood by the following 2 × 2 table:

Screening Test	Result	Diagnosis	Total
	Disease	Normal	
Positive	a	b	$a + b$
	True Positive	False Positive	
Negative	c	d	$c + d$
	False Negative	True negative	
Total	$a + c$	$b + d$	$a + b + c + d$

a = True positive = Those who have the disease and the test result is also positive

b = False positive = Those who do not have the disease but the test result is positive

c = False negative = Those who have the disease but the test is negative

d = True negative = Those who have no disease and the test is also negative

$a/(a + b) \times 100$ = **Predictive value of positive test:** Probability of an individual really having the disease, if the test result is positive.

$d/(c + d) \times 100$ = **Predictive value of a negative test:** Probability of an individual really not having disease, if the test result is negative.

$c/(a + c) \times 100 =$ **Percentage of false negative**

Percentage of non-disease persons wrongly diagnosed as having disease–Positive test.

$b/(b + d) \times 100 =$ **Percentage of false positive.**

Percentage of disease persons wrongly identified as not having disease–Negative test.

Sensitivity–$a/(a + c)$ – Ability of a test to correctly identify those having the disease

Specificity–$d/(b + d)$ – Ability of a test to correctly identify those not having the disease.

Example

A new screening test for any disease has been launched. It was administered in 1000 persons, 135 out of which are known to have the disease. The test was positive in 110 of the persons with the disease as well as in 45 persons without the disease. Evaluate the screening test by all the measures given in Table 8.2.

Table 8.2: Screening test result

Result	Diagnosis		Total
	Diseased	Non diseased	
Positive	110 (a)	45 (b)	155 (a + b)
Negative	25 (c)	820 (d)	845 (c + d)
Total	135 (a + c)	865 (b + d)	1000 (a + b + c + d)

Answers

1. Sensitivity (true positive)

   $a/a + c \times 100 = 110/110 + 25 \times 100 = 110/135 \times 100 = 81.48\%$

2. Specificity (true negative)

   $b/b + d \times 100 = 820/820 + 45 \times 100 = 94.79\%$

3. Predictive value of a positive test

   $a/a + b \times 100 = 110/110 + 45 \times 100 = 70.96\%$

4. Predictive value of a negative test

   $d/c + d \times 100 = 820/820 + 25 \times 100 = 97.04\%$

5. False positive

   $b/b + d \times 100 = 45/45 + 820 \times 100 = 5.20\%$

6. False negative

   $c/a + c \times 100 = 25/25 + 110 \times 100 = 18.51\%$

7. Prevalence of disease

   $a + c/a + b + c + d = 110 + 25/110 + 25 + 45 + 820 \times 100 = 13.5\%$

9

Association and Causation

The ultimate aim of epidemiological studies is to discover the cause of disease, so that the disease is prevented or controlled. The understanding of cause of disease is important in health field, not only for prevention but also in diagnosis and the application of correct treatment.

Descriptive epidemiology identify disease problem and relates disease to host, agent and environment, while analytic and interventional epidemiology confirm or refute the observed association between cause and effect.

In epidemiology a cause is an event, condition, characteristic or combination of these factors which play an important role in producing the disease. It simply means that cause must precede a disease or other way we can say that disease cannot develop in its absence.

Epidemiology proceeds from demonstration of statistical association to demonstration that the association is causal.

Association does not always mean that it is causal. Statistically we are having so many tests of significance (t-test, chi-square test, z-test, etc.) which can give the result that the association is significant, but ultimately the aim is to prove the association being causal.

Association can be of following types:

- Spurious association
- Indirect association
- Direct association

SPURIOUS ASSOCIATION

Spurious association is mostly observed when there is selection bias. The two groups, which are going to be compared, are not properly matched. As in a study of UK, it was found that perinatal mortality is more among hospital deliveries and conclusion was drawn that home is a safer place for deliveries. But it is not true. The deliveries which are conducted at hospitals are mostly high risk cases. So here high risk cases are compared with the normal cases and thus there chances of having a spurious association when matching is not proper.

INDIRECT ASSOCIATION

It is mostly observed where confounding factor is present, i.e. a common factor influencing both the groups under observation.

As it was observed that goiter is present at high altitude as compared to other areas and the conclusions drawn was, altitude is having association with goiter. It seems correct also. But when it was compared with group of people at the same altitude having goiter and no goiter, or compared with goiter patients of low altitude, then it was found wrong. Then it was noticed that goiter is linked with intake of iodine not with the high altitude, of course, which is less available at high altitude. So it is an indirect association.

Direct association: It is one to one relationship factor. A is directly related to affect B. It was Koch's postulate in germ theory which led to formulation that, i.e.

• The organism must be present in every case of disease
• The organism must be able to be isolated and grown in pure culture
• The organism must, when inoculated into a suspected animal, cause the specific disease
• The organism must, then be recovered from the animal and identified

This concept of disease causation/association was demonstrated in anthrax, but does not fit well in many diseases as:

• Many causes are operating
• In some, the causative agent may disappear after the disease development.
• It is observed in tuberculosis, that *Mycobacterium tuberculosis* is the necessary cause, but other components are also equally important for causation of disease.

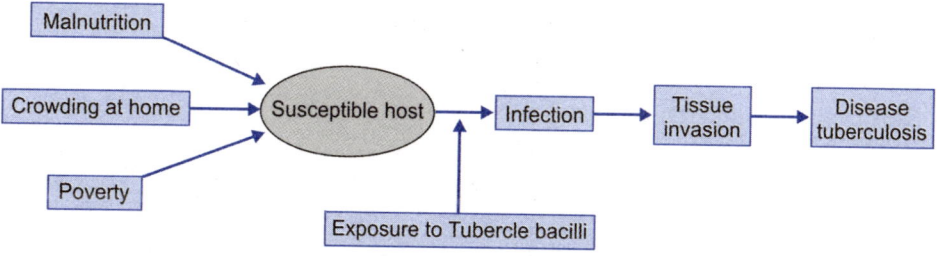

It has also been observed that single cause or factor may lead to more than one outcome, as a case of hemolytic streptococci, which can present as streptococcal tonsillitis, scarlet fever or erysipelas.

In this way one to one causal relationship is not sufficient to explain these type of conditions, where we should apply multi-factorial etiology of disease, as already explained for TB.

FACTORS IN CAUSATION

Four types of factors play part in disease causation and all are necessary

• Predisposing factors – create state of susceptibility, e.g. age, sex, previous illness, etc.

- Enabling factors – favor the development of disease, e.g. low income, poor nutrition, bad housing, etc.
- Precipitating factors – associated with onset of a disease, e.g. disease agent or noxious agent.
- Reinforcing factors – aggravate the established disease, e.g. repeated exposure, unduly hard work.

All these factors, in common are described under the heading 'risk factors', which are having positive association with risk of development of a disease.
Epidemiological studies can measure the relative contribution of each factor to disease occurrence and corresponding potential reduction in disease from the elimination of each risk factor.

GUIDELINES FOR ESTABLISHING THE CAUSE OF A DISEASE

As it has been already explained that association is not always causal, also the single aspect cannot lead us to a conclusion about causal relation. There are guidelines for establishing the cause and as many guidelines favor the relationship, it is more in favor of causal relationship.

Before an association is assessed for the possibility that it is causal, other explanations, such as chance, bias and confounding factors have to be excluded.

The steps are

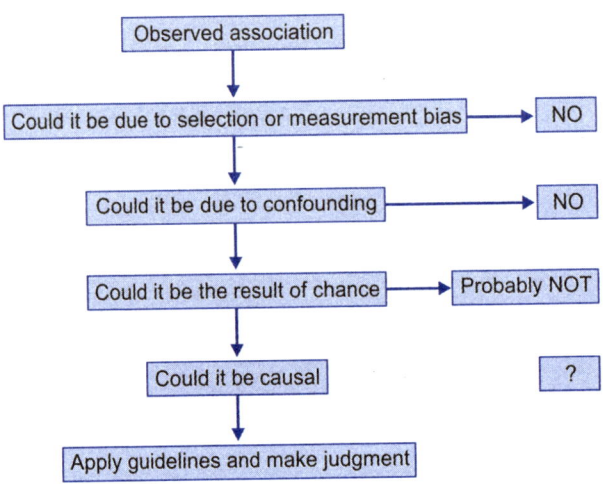

GUIDELINES FOR CAUSAL RELATIONSHIP

These are following guidelines which must be tested in sequence and then conclusion should be drawn:
1. Temporal association
2. Biological plausibility
3. Consistency
4. Strength
5. Specificity of association
6. Dose–response relationship
7. Coherence

8. Reversibility
9. Study design

1. **Temporal Relationship:** It is important and crucial that the cause must precede the effect. It is usually self-evident in acute diseases, e.g. water and food borne outbreaks, but in chronic diseases it is difficult to know or we can say, difficulties may arise in case control or cross-sectional studies when measurement of cause and effect are made at same time and effect may in fact change the exposure. Of course, the repeated measurement of exposure at more than one point in time and different location may strengthen the evidence, as it is observed in cohort and interventional studies.

2. **Biological Plausibility:** It means that there is explanation of changes occurring at cellular level after the stimuli (exposure or agent or factor). It is evident that after inhalation of smoke into lungs after cigarette smoking, there is deposition of chemical carcinogen like tar, carbon monoxide, nicotine. Tar is related to carcinogenic changes. So smoking has a biologically plausible association with carcinoma lung. Increasing doses (no. of cigarettes per day and for long duration) leading to increased incidence indicates biological gradient. It should also be kept in mind that lack of plausibility may simply reflect lack of medical knowledge.

3. **Consistency:** It is demonstrated by several studies giving the same result. This is particularly important when varieties of designs are used in different settings. Of course, when the results of several studies are being interpreted the best designed ones should be given more weightage or result can be interpreted by meta-analysis.

4. **Strength:** This is measured by size of risk ratio that is relative risk or odds ratio (OR). Higher the values, greater is the likelihood of causal association, e.g. cigarette smokers have approximately two fold increase in the risk of acute MI as compared to non-smokers. The risk of lung cancer in smokers as compared with non-smokers has been shown in various studies to be increased between 10 to 20 times higher.

5. **Specificity of Association:** We have learnt in Koch's postulates about germ theory, where one germ was producing a specific disease. But in most of the cases it is not applicable.

   Simply talking about smoking and lung cancer, the disease is not only caused by cigarette smoking, it can also be due to air pollution especially asbestos or other hazards. Similarly smoking not only produces lung cancer but also results in heart disease, bronchitis, peptic ulcer, etc. So it does not give a clear clue but also does not rule out its causal relationship.

   Attributable risk is one, which can be estimated for this relevance. Smoking of cigarettes attributes 80 to 90 % in causation of lung cancer.

6. **Dose–response Relationship:** A dose response relationship occurs when changes in the level of a possible cause are associated with changes in the prevalence or incidence of the effect. It has been clearly demonstrated that number of cigarettes and duration of smoking have causal relationship between exposure or dose and disease.

7. **Coherence:** This is the criteria which demonstrate coherence with known factors that are thought to be relevant, e.g. increased per capita cigarette consumption and increase in incidence of lung cancer is coherent.

8. **Reversibility:** When the removal of possible cause results in a reduced incidence of disease, the association being causal is strengthened as in case of smoking. If smoking

is reduced, the risk of lung cancer is lowered as compared to people who continue to smoke. It is not true for all cases, as in HIV and AIDS if the virus has entered once, and the harmful practice is stopped, even then the irreversible changes continue to occur.

9. **Study Design:** The ability of study design to prove causation is a most important consideration. It can be summarized as:

Type of study	Ability to prove causation
Randomized controlled trials	Strong
Cohort studies	Moderate plus
Case control studies	moderate
Cross sectional/ecological	weak

CONCLUSION ABOUT ESTABLISHING THE CAUSE

We have discussed so many criteria, but no single criteria can definitely or conclusively provide the idea that associates is causal.

The conclusion should be drawn on the basis of evidence. As we have discussed, the temporal association is not always possible, dose response and reversibility criteria is not applicable in all situations. The gap in our knowledge may be a hindrance to explain the plausibility. The likelihood of a causal relationship is increased, when many different criteria lead to same conclusion.

10

Investigation of an Epidemic

An epidemiologist is often required to investigate an outbreak of disease in his area. The main purpose to investigate the outbreak is to control the outbreak and prevent future occurrence of disease/outbreak with the application of knowledge gained from investigations.

AIM OF INVESTIGATION

a. To confirm that an outbreak exists.
b. Describe the epidemic according to the variables of person, place and time.
c. Establish the source of agent, its mode of transmission and vehicle/ vector they may be involved.
d. Identify susceptible populations that are at a higher risk.
e. Take measure to contain the epidemic.
f. Report the procedure of investigation to appropriate authority.

STEPS IN EPIDEMIOLOGICAL INVESTIGATION

- Verification of diagnosis.
- Confirmation about the existence of an epidemic.
- Description of epidemic.
- Assessment of environmental conditions including entomological and zoonotic conditions depending upon the nature of outbreak.
- Laboratory confirmation, if possible.
- Formulation of hypothesis about the possible source and method of transmission.
- Management and control of the outbreak.
- Documentation of the outbreak.

1. **Verification of Diagnosis:** Whenever there is an outbreak, initial responsibility is to confirm the diagnosis. In most of the instances, it has to be done on clinical grounds in cases, where laboratory confirmation is needed or is easily available, one should do that.

2. **Confirmation of the Existence of the Epidemic:** It is confirmed by studying the records available related to the disease which is to be confirmed. It can be obtained from other institutions and survey reports available. One may also be required to

study records pertaining to disease which closely resemble the diagnosis in the present situation.

Often the comparison is not necessary as in common source epidemic such as acute gastroenteritis, food poisoning, etc.

3. **Description of an Epidemic:** To describe the epidemic, the information about the cases is required, which is not only available in form of reported cases, but one have to visit the area affected to collect information.

For this purpose, a questionnaire can also be prepared, so that any relevant information is not missed.

The information must be collected in reference to time, place and person.

Time distribution is studied by making a table, according the onset of symptoms and then curve (graph) can be drawn.

The shape of the curve helps to know the type of the epidemic.

- The sudden rise and sudden fall of the epidemic curve indicates 'common source', i.e. single exposure epidemic
- Sudden rise and gradual fall of the epidemic curve indicates 'common source' but in repeated exposure epidemic.
- Gradual rise and gradual fall of the epidemic curve indicates propagated epidemic.

• Place distribution can be studied by plotting map of geographical area. This pictorial presentation shows at glance. Rapid search is made by the area health workers by door to door survey to detect new cases. This should be carried out every day till the area declared free of epidemic. This period is taken as twice the incubation period of disease, since the occurrence of last case in the area of high and low density. This further gives a clue about source of infection and even the mode of spread

• Person distribution of epidemic is studied by collecting the following data

- Total population of the area
- Total number of persons being affected
- Total number of deaths, if any
- Age and sexwise, according to occupation and social class distribution of the disease.
- After collection of relevant data, define the population at risk, calculate the attack rate, death rate, incubation period, source and spread of infection

4. **Assessment of Environmental Conditions:** Environmental condition which include physical, chemical, biological and social environments are then assessed to find out a clue to the factors involving transmission.

In addition metrological information, status of water supply and sewage disposal are collected and laboratory findings are also obtained in relation to these sources.

If the outbreak is suspected to be vector borne, study various entomological indices and try to isolate causative organism from the agent identified.

5. **Laboratory Investigations:** Samples for laboratory examination are collected from active patients, carriers, vectors and zoonotic reservoirs and the other sources like water, food, soil, etc. as the case may be.

For virological studies, special transport media and cold chain are available and for bacteriological studies simple media are used.

The quantity of the sample should be sufficient for carrying out all the necessary tests.

6. **Formulation of Hypothesis:** After all information is available, now a hypothesis is formulated in terms of diagnosis, causative agent, possible source of infection, mode of spread, environmental factors favoring the occurrence of epidemic.

   This can be unifocal or multifocal. It should also be kept in mind that the outbreak of disease is the result of interaction between agent, host and environment. Thus, it is necessary to link all these factors to confirm the hypothesis.

   The hypothesis, thus formed should be tested by calculating exposure rate. If the exposure rate is more among the cases than among control, then there is association between suspected factor and the disease.

7. **Management and Control of the Outbreak:** Control of the outbreak will vary from disease to disease, however, the aim of any control measure is to break the chain of transmission.

   The recommendation to control the outbreak is:

   1. Short term–for current outbreak

   2. Long term–to avoid such outbreak in future

   These measures can be:

   - Elimination of reservoir
   - Breaking the chain of transmission, i.e. isolation, quarantine, etc.
   - Protection of susceptibles by immunizing agent or by improvement of quality of life.

8. **Documentation of the Epidemic:** Immediately after the investigation, a report has to be prepared for submission to the health authorities. The report should have the following components:

   a. Preamble

   b. Description of the outbreak

   c. Methods of investigation

   d. Analysis and interpretation of findings

   e. Recommendations

   If the investigation is expected to take quite some time, a short preliminary report highlighting the nature of outbreak and control measure recommended may be submitted and this may be followed up by a detailed report incorporating all relevant information.

EPIDEMIC CHARACTERISTICS IN GENERAL AND SOME SPECIAL CHARACTERISTICS OF COMMON OUTBREAK

One should, however, keep in mind that no two outbreaks are exactly the same. Each disease has its special characteristics. As such, sufficiently detailed instructions cannot be suggested which will apply in every instance. But there are certain fundamentals which, if followed should result in a successful investigation and one will be able to determine the circumstances leading to the outbreak and obtain information, which one may use to prevent a recurrence. The steps to be followed have already been enumerated. One must also remember that very often, one will get only one opportunity to collect facts, which may point to the cause of the outbreak. Ordinarily, it is not possible or practicable to return to the same place or interview the same individuals several times for information, which could have been collected earlier. As such, one will have to follow the prescribed procedure, when one undertakes any investigation.

Special characteristics of some common outbreaks: outbreaks which you likely to handle as medical officer at PHC.

Water Borne Outbreaks

I. It is confined to those individuals who are drinking water from a particular source.

II. It is co-existence with the distribution of supply.

III. It affects all age and sex groups who use that water.

IV. The outbreak is usually explosive.

V. The outbreak stops after stoppage of use of that water. It is used after disinfection of water.

VI. The outbreak may be seasonal.

VII. The contaminant can be detected by laboratory examination.

Food Borne Outbreaks

These may be caused by a toxic substance or through infection by organisms. An outbreak due to food poisoning has the following features:

I. Sudden onset with sudden cessation.

II. Occurs within a few hours after a common meal taken by a group of people, family members, etc.

III. Is associated with vomiting and purging.

IV. Non users escape.

V. All age and sex groups consuming suspected food suffer.

VI. Severity depending on quantity consumed.

VII. Particular item of food can be traced.

VIII. Bacteriological evidence detectable except for toxin.

Vector Borne Outbreaks

I. Cases geographically distributed to the areas where vector is available.

II. Seasonal variation corresponds to the growth and density of vector species.

III. All age and sex groups usually suffer.

IV. Epidemic comes down with decrease in vector density.

V. Parasite can be detected in the vector.

VI. Outbreak can be controlled by controlling the vector, sanitation etc. as the case may be.

Outbreak due to Droplet Infection

I. This may have explosive rise as in influenza Assuming normalcy after some time, or it may have a slow progress as in tuberculosis.

II. Droplet infections are usually associated with overcrowding, poor hygienic environment, etc. in case of diphtheria, depending upon the contact, there is a slow fall.

III. A similar nature is exhibited by mumps.

IV. Both diphtheria and mumps may assume epidemic proportion particularly in residential schools, hostels, etc. where considerable overcrowding exists.

V. Age distribution is different according to disease, but younger age groups are more vulnerable.

11

Selection of Research Problem: A Major Step in Epidemiology

A research problem is a question that a researcher wants to answer or solve. Every problem which comes to the mind or even suggested by an experienced person may not fit to be a good research problem.

Selection of a research problem depends on researcher's knowledge, skills, interest, expertise, motivation and creativity with respect to the subject of enquiry.

Research problem is defined as "a problem which can be an interrogative sentence or statement that asks what relation exists between two or more variables". The answer to question will provide what is sought in the research.

COMPONENTS OF RESEARCH PROBLEM

Any research problem has six components:
1. Relevance of the study
2. Title of the study
3. Operational definitions of the variables
4. Delimitations of the study
5. Objectives of the study
6. Scope and limitations of the study

IDENTIFICATION OF RESEARCH PROBLEM

It is the first and most important step in the research process. Generally a broad area is selected and in the next step, broad topic is delimited/narrowed and ultimately specific one sentence statement of the problem is selected.

As to begin with, the researcher thinks about reproductive period of women, then nutrition during reproductive period and ultimately it is limited to assessment of iron deficiency in women during their reproductive period, i.e. 15 – 49 years of age.

SOURCES OF RESEARCH PROBLEM

There are various resources which initiate the idea for research. Few important sources are as follows:
1. Personal experience and area of interest
2. Field or clinical experience

3. Review of literature and existing research
4. Social issues of the society
5. Active discussion with experts
6. Previous research for further analysis

These are various sources but there are also various stages which one experiences in life.

Personal interest in a particular area inspires the person to search more about the field and certainly one go to consult the literature available. On the other hand, while reviewing literature, some new field is found, and one gets interested to search in detail about it.

While working at the place of job, the experience also provocate to go in depth about the areas which still need exploration or new idea originated out of practical work. There may be some difficulties or novel way to perform the work.

One may be vigilant about the events occurring in the society. Every day the new issues are coming up with challenge and new problems are posed and one wants to get their scientific answers. These social issues may be rape, drug addiction, effect of unemployment, aspirations of youth, increasing suicide and road traffic accidents, etc.

As we go through literature, similarly having a brain storming discussion with the experts also provide some insight to explore the areas which are unanswered.

The researcher starts with one area, limited aspect of that area and after completion, researcher feels that there are other aspects which are as important to be explored.

So in this way, person with an inquisitive mind always remain interested to know new aspects and wherever it is possible through survey or in a scientific methodology, one can proceed in this direction.

CRITERIA FOR SELECTION OF A GOOD RESEARCH PROBLEM

There are few important aspects which must be kept in mind during selection of research problem:
1. Significance to the community and profession
2. New and unique
3. Feasible to carry out
4. Availability of subjects/volunteers
5. Administrative and support of colleagues
6. Researchers competence
7. Ethical consideration
8. Problem solving outcome.

A MAJOR STEP IN RESEARCH

Research may be defined as an investigation undertaken in order to discover new facts, get additional information, etc. The important characteristics of research are:
1. It is based on observable experience or empirical evidence.
2. It demands accurate observation and description.
3. The goal is to discover cause and effective relationship.
4. It gives beyond the specific objects, groups situations and emphasizes the development of generalization principals or theories.

5. It is objective and logical. The research should eliminate personal bias. The attempt is to testing rather than proving.
6. It is directed towards the solution of a problem.

Stages in Research

1. Formulation of the research problem
2. Study of related literature
3. Development of hypothesis
4. Preparing research design
5. Methodology or strategy
6. Preparation of research report

1. Formulation of the Research Problem

The research should begin with a statement of problem. First, the researcher has to identify and select a research problem. The noun, 'Problem', has conventional and technical meaning. In the conventional sense, a problem is a set of conditions needing discussion, a decision, a solution or information. A research problem implies the possibility of empirical investigation, i.e. of data collection and analysis.

A research problem in contrast with a practical problem is formally stated to indicate a need for investigation.

Qualitative research problem are phrased as research statements or questions but never as hypothesis.

A research hypothesis implies deductive reasoning, whereas, qualitative research uses primarily inductive reasoning to suggest an understanding of a particular situation.

Quantitative problem states the situation or context in such a way as to limit the problem.

2. Study of Related Literature

A careful review of related literature is one of the major steps in any research study. The literature review enables a researcher to gain further insight into the purpose and results of a study.

There are many sources to review the relevant literature, i.e. journals, reports, books, monographed government documents and dissertations, etc.

Related literature is obviously relevant to the problem such as previous research investigates the same variables or similar question, reference to the theory and empirical testing of the theory and studies of similar practices.

A study of related literature must precede any well planned research. A review of literature saves served purpose in research. It enables the researchers to:
- Define and limit the problem
- Place the study in a historical and associated perspective
- Avoid unintentional and unnecessary replication
- Select promising methods and measures
- Relate the findings to previous knowledge and suggest further research

3. Development of Hypothesis

Hypothesis may be defined as a tentative proposition suggested as a solution to a problem. It is a suggested solution to a problem, which is later tested by an investigator.

'Bar' and 'Scates' defined hypothesis as a statement temporarily accepted as true in light of what is at the time known about a phenomenon and it is employed as a basis for action in the search for new truth. We can understand that a hypothesis is a statement of a potential empirical relationship between two or more variable and also it is possible to determine whether a hypothesis is probably true or false. Uses/purpose of hypothesis are:

- It provides tentative explanation and facilitates thinking process
- It provides related statement that can be directly tested in a study
- It helps to keep the study in limits.
- It provides the frame work for reporting the conclusions

4. Preparing Research Design

The function of a research is to preview a plan for collection of relevant evidence with minimal expenditure of efforts, time and money. Usually research designs can be as cross-section of, i.e. descriptive, explorative or analyze and experimentation or interventional. Hence, depending on the purpose any one of these may be selected as research design.

5. Methodolgy/Strategy

This indicates the method in which the investigator is going to conduct the research and includes the following parts:

a. *Sample*: The population/universe from which the sample for study has to be taken is defined. After that, next is to calculate the sample size, keeping in view the prevalence of the problem (disease). And lastly, the method of sampling to be used should also be clearly mentioned. Random to purposive sampling, there are many sampling techniques.

b. *Collection of data*: The collection of appropriate data for any research problem is very essential. There are several ways of collecting the data. Usually primary data can be collected through experiments or survey. In the survey, the data is collected though a tool, i.e. a good questionnaire which is also known as 'instrument'.

c. *Analysis of data:* After collection the data should be tabulated and analyzed. The suitable statistical techniques may be planned well in advance. Hence, the researcher can analyze the collected data with the help of various statistical measures.

d. *Hypothesis testing:* After analysis of data the hypothesis should be tested using t-test, z-test, F-test, correlation, etc. This leads to either accepting or rejecting the hypothesis.

e. *Generalization and interpretation:* If the hypothesis is tested and upheld several times, it may be possible for the researcher to derive generalization. On the basis of co-relational analysis the data is interpreted in term of cause and effect or strength of association.

6. Preparation of Research Report

Finally the researcher has to prepare the report of what has been done by him. In the research report, the researcher should write the following things:

- Introduction
- Review of literature
- Aim and objectives
- Observation and discussion
- Summary and conclusion
- Recommendations
- Bibliography

Hence, in any scientific investigation, the above stages should be clearly planned, so that we can conduct the research in a systematic manner.

TOOLS OF RESEARCH

In most of the research survey, especially in large sample size or multicentric research survey, many investigators or field staff workers are required. The first and most essential requirement of collection of data is uniformity of data.

It has been observed that mostly there are biases in data collection, related to instrument or usage of tools.

In case of field study, the question as a tool is most frequently used tool. Now-a-days, there are standard tools prepared by expert agencies like WHO, UNICEF or other specialists of that field. But it is also a practice that researcher or principal investigator has to construct his own tool.

The frequently used methods in public health or clinical investigations are:

1. Observations
2. Interviews
3. Questionnaire
4. Rating scales

Before employing the tools or test, we should ensure the following important criteria of a test:

1. Reliability
2. Validity
3. Easy administration and interpretation
4. Economical

While constructing an instrument or tool, researcher should follow few basic steps:

- Write out specific objective for your instrument, as there is objective to assess knowledge, attitude and practice towards breast feeding.
- There should be separate and specific approach for knowledge assessed professionals who are expert in the assessed area to review the items.
- Revise if necessary, find a small sample of individuals that is similar to those that will be used in actual study and administer the instrument to them. It is called 'Pilot study'.
- Check the clarity, ambiguity in sentences, time for completion that may have been experienced.
- Check for an adequate distribution of scores for each item in the instrument, i.e. there should be an opportunity for responding to both the extremes (poor to excellent).
- Revise, delete and add items where necessary, depending upon the feedback from pilot study. Two main types of tools are discussed in detail.

I. Interview

It is one of the important and powerful tool for data collection in social and medical case history of patient, is an example of interview.

It is mostly a verbal method but it is not only the words spoken which matters but also the gesture, facial expressions, pauses, modification of voices, etc. also matter in the interview. So one expert opinion is an effective informal verbal and non-verbal conversation.

All interviews have three elements in common:

1. A person to person relationship.
2. A mean of communication with each other.
3. Awareness on the part of at least one of the persons for the purpose of interview.
   Following steps are involved in interviewing:
   - Preparation of interview and establishing rapport.
   - The unfolding of the problem.
   - The joint working out of the problem.
   - The closing of the interview.
   - Evaluation of the interview.
   - Follow up of the interview.

While expecting an interview, the researcher should be friendly and courteous to keep the respondent at ease. No sign of surprise or disapproval should be shown because it may embarrass the respondent. If some questions are misunderstood or complex, they should be repeated and paraphrased.

While collecting the response the interviewer should write down the actual words of the respondent. It should not be polished or corrected. It should be recorded in verbatim (as spoken).

Merits

1. It is the most dynamic way of understanding the individual as a whole.
2. It is relatively easy to conduct.
3. It is very useful in those cases where the individual is illiterate.
4. It is usually explorative and at that movement, while talking some new ideas or questions can emerge out of conversation.

Demerits

1. It is very expensive as visiting people at different places involve many kind of expenses as well as time.
2. Sometimes the respondent may give biased response.
3. It requires high level of expertise. The investigator should possess qualities of objectivity, insight and sensitivity.
4. Generalization of the information is also difficult.

II. Questionnaire

It is a research tool containing a set of questions to be answered by the respondent.

Questions are useful

- When people cannot be personally contacted.
- When we cannot personally interview so many respondents.

These can be:
1. Structured questionnaire
2. Non-structured questionnaire
   Structured questionnaire contains definite and concrete questions and non-structured questionnaire are open ended and whatsoever response one feels, the respondent is free to mention. Non-structured questionnaire are mainly used in qualitative studies like in social sciences or research into social aspects of disease.

These also can be divided into
1. *Open ended*, i.e. interviewee is free to express and observer should note, whatsoever subject is telling.
2. *Close ended*, i.e. in which options to be ticked are alredy mentined like; yes/No.

Construction of a questionnaire

- It includes important items only.
- Responses expected are simple, say in form of yes or no.
- It should not be suggestive, as "do you see laughter channel", it should be "which TV channel you watch?" and similarly "whether you eat green leafy vegetables?", say "what do you eat in a day".
- It should not embarrass the respondent.
- It should be clearly worded.

Characteristics of a good questionnaire

1. All questions are relevant and significant, i.e. focusing on the topic.
2. It seeks information which cannot be procured by any other mode, i.e. it seeks information not available from other sources.
3. It is short but complete.
4. The questions are objective but directions are clear.
5. The items are categorically arranged.
6. The order of presentation of questions item should be logical.
7. They can be tabulated and interpreted.
8. They should not be ambiguous, i.e. meaning conveyed to every respondent should be similar.

Problems in preparing questionnaire

1. Leading questions (No place for these)
2. Cross checking (should be avoided)
3. Length of the questionnaire
4. Limitations of responses
5. Types of questions (open and closed ended)
6. Categories and there place of order in sequence
7. Short gun questions?

Advantages

1. Less expensive
2. Less time consuming
3. No technical skill is required to administer.
4. Large number can be consulted at one time.

PART II

Biostatistics

12

Data and its Types

When you can measure what you are speaking about and express it in numbers, you know something about it but when you cannot measure it, when you cannot express it in numbers, your knowledge is of meager and unsatisfactory kind.

— Lord Kelvin

Expressing in terms of numbers provides a better sense of understanding. India is a poor country have no sense and similarly every body is having mobile phone these days is also not a scientific expression. When we say these days diabetes is rampant, every body complains of high blood pressure are also vague expressions. On one side India is a developing country and the world's richest person is in India, on the other hand one-third people of this country living below poverty line. Statistics gives us a more realistic picture. Even a simple numerical statement has a limited value. When we say per capita income of India is ₹ 20,000 per year, it doesn't clarify the sense that India is a poor country unless we do not clarify that USA is having 15 times higher per capita income than India. Then it qualifies the statement that on this basis we say that India is a poor country. So, in this way statistics is not simply a numerical expression but even wider then that. Science of Medicine is not a pure science as physics, chemistry and mathematics. It is the art and science where there are always chances of empirical expression.

When we talk about statistics in Medicine, our focus is to establish strength of association or giving a credit to some factors responsible for that event. But we must remember that statistics is one of the tools, apart from many others. There are guidelines for causation, i.e. biological plausibility, temporal association, type of study undertaken by investigator, etc. and out of these guidelines one is statistically associated or statistically significant result.

Quantification is the one factor or measurement of even qualities that has made possible to understand the mental and social phenomenon. We can provide a rank to even beauty.

Today, if social sciences like sociology, psychology, and anthropology are considered under the discipline of science, the reason is that the quality of any expression can be quantified. We can provide rank to even beauty, work capacity, social status, etc. similarly mental phenomenon can also be expressed in numbers and can undergo further statistical analysis. In this way statistics is one of the tools in the hand of researchers for predicting his results.

STATISTICS

It is a science of numbers. Biostatistics on the other hand is number applied to living persons. It is different from mathematics which is purely a number game applied to each and every aspect.

Here it must be understood that why as a medical man we need statistics. First and foremost is, that we as a medical faculty always talk about numbers when we measure pulse rate, respiratory rate or blood pressure or even when we count red blood cells, platelets or even biochemicals present. After counting or measuring we conclude or interpret it as in normal or beyond normal range. It is obvious that for comparison we need normal. Who gives us normal value or normal range? It is statistics, which provides us **limits of normalcy**.

Normal values lead us to comparison. This comparison may be with in the two pockets of the same area or it may be interstate or international comparison. It is the comparison that gives us an insight that the difference between the two means is due to chance or natural variation or some external factors playing a role.

Moreover, statistics give us a number, which is the frequency of a particular event (disease, death, accidents, etc.) and in a way, provides us the magnitude of that event. Magnitude is a way to reflect the situation and stress upon effective planning. Planning needs monitoring and evaluation, which requires data for comparison of results for implementation. Therefore, we can say that statistics deals with techniques or methods of collection of data, classification, summarizing, interpretation, drawing inferences, testing of hypothesis and making recommendations.

A comprehensive definition by Prof Harace Secrist: "Statistics are aggregates of facts affected to marked extent by multiplicity of causes, numerically expressed, enumerated or estimated according to reasonable standards of accuracy, collected in a systematic manner for a predetermined purpose and placed in relation to each other."

As a medical person, it must be remembered that, for us statistics is not a game of numbers or fun game. While collecting data, presenting and analyzing, it should always be kept in mind that our aim is to draw some valid conclusion. We should always look for inferences, based on which some solid planning can be done to relieve the humanity from sickness. All statistics are numerical statements of facts, but all numerical statements of facts are not statistics.

SEQUENCE IN BIOSTATISTICS

Statistical methods mainly fall into two broad categories:
i. Descriptive statistics and
ii. Inferential statistics
i. Descriptive statistics as the name indicates simply describe or summarize data (mean or average height of girls of twenty years or ratio of male to female children below six years).
ii. Inferential statistics as the name indicates, deals with 'making inferences' means it goes beyond the actual data. It helps in generating the results after having observed only a sample.

Flow chart of sequence of biostatstics

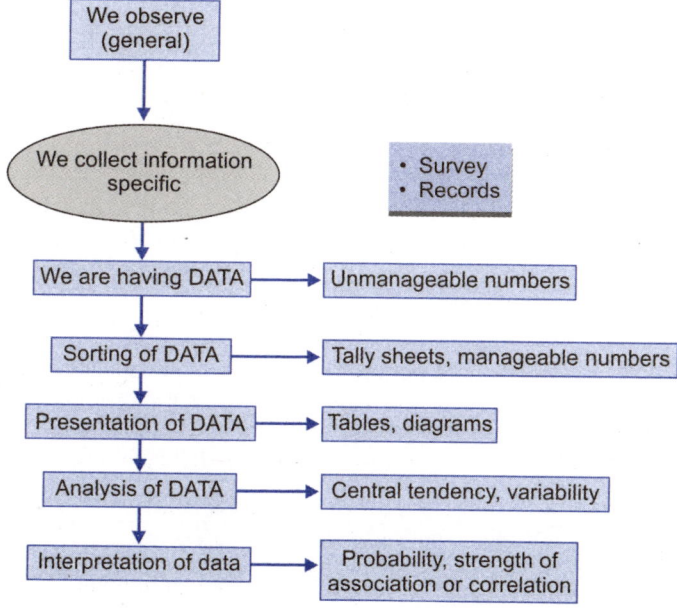

DATA

This is measured or counted facts expressed in figures. It is divided into two broad categories:

    a. Qualitative data (or discrete data) and

    b. Quantitative data (or continuous data)

a. Qualitative Data (Discrete Data)

They are obtained by counting the individuals having the same characteristic or attribute and not by measurement as the characteristic or attribute cannot be measured.

    We can say there is only one variable, i.e. number of persons, i.e. persons with same characteristics are counted to form specific groups or classes.

    For example, after a particular vaccination say measles, out of 200 children, only 15 were attacked and on the other hand 75 children had attack of measles, who were from unvaccinated group. Here the characteristic or attribute, i.e. attacked by the disease remains the same but the frequency of persons (attacked or not attacked) varies.

    Qualitative data are discrete or discontinuous in nature as values of various items cannot be divided, i.e. number of persons having different blood groups, i.e. there is one characteristic for one whole group or class, i.e. no split is there. There are four types of blood groups A, B, O, AB. There is nothing in between. There is characteristic like married or unmarried, nothing like half-married. If, we say there are widows or widowers, then there is another characteristic, which we have to add but that is again a discrete character.

b. Quantitative Data (Continuous Data)

In comparison to qualitative data, they have magnitude. The characteristic is measured either on interval scale or ratio scale. This type of data is classified on two scales, i.e. characteristic or variable and frequency. Here the characteristic is given the name variable as it varies. In qualitative data the characteristic does not vary. It is married or unmarried but in height measurement, the data varies. As height varies from person to person, similarly, hemoglobin varies from person to person. It varies from sex and age point of view also. Thus, we find the characteristic as well as frequency both vary from person to person. It is continuous because characteristic and frequency are subdivided due to range.

For example: The height of 100 students of one class of was measured. Its range was found to be from 150 cm to 162 cm. While making the groups on interval scale, it was seen that from 150 to 152 cm, there were ten students; 153 to 155 cm there were 15 students and so on. Thus, we find that characteristics as well as the frequency vary from person to person as well as from group to group.

Table 12.1: Difference between qualitative and quantitative data

Qualitative data	Quantitative data
Discrete data	Continuous data
No subgroup	Subgroup split
One attribute	Variables
No magnitude	Measured on interval or ratio scale
Statistical method employed on such data are SEP and Chi-square test	Statistical methods employed on such data are mean, standard deviation, coefficient of variation, correlation coefficient

Table 12.2: Examples of various types of data

Type of variable	Variable	Categories
Qualitative	Sex	Male, Female
	Status	Upper/lower class
	Religion	Hindu/Sikh
Quantitative	Age	1 day to 100 years
	Height	50 cm to 200 cm
	Income	₹ 50 to ₹ 500/day

Collection of Data

Depending upon the source, data is of two types: (a) Primary (b) Secondary.

a. **Primary data:** It is original data collected and recorded by investigators. This is first hand information. This is collected by:

   i. Surveys

  ii. Experiments

Surveys: This is a way of collection of data actively and with planning. This is carried out in the field by trained teams, mostly for epidemiological studies.

Surveys provide rate, ratios, incidence, prevalence and we can apply statistical tests on data to draw some useful inferences.

Experiments: These are performed in the laboratories of physiology, biochemistry, pharmacology and hospital wards (may be medicine, surgery, orthopedics, anesthesia, etc.) Experiments provide mainly comparison data on different clinical trials or laboratory investigations.

Mode of Collection of Primary Data

- Direct personal investigation
- Indirect oral investigation
- Information through correspondents
- Information through mailed questionnaire
- Questionnaire through interviewer

Direct Personal Investigation

Investigators collect data personally. Investigator has to meet person concerned and take interview and collect the information.

Indirect oral Investigation

Under this method, the investigator collects the facts by interviewing persons not those from whom information is to be collected instead he makes contacts with some other persons who are directly or indirectly in touch with them (subjects).

Information through Correspondents

In this case, investigator appoints local or correspondents in different field of enquiry. They collect and send the required information and investigator ultimately processes the data.

Information through Mailed Questionnaire

In this method, a questionnaire (a list of question to be asked) is sent to the informants by post.

Questionnaire through Interviewer

Here, information is collected on the basis of a questionnaire through the interviewer. He fills the question himself by asking questions to interviewee.

ESSENTIALS OF GOOD QUESTIONNAIRE

- Questions should be simple and clear in order
- Questions should be small as far as possible
- Questions should be properly arranged. Simple formal questions and then other questions
- Preferably Yes and No option questions should be framed
- Cross check questions be included
- Question should be directly related to investigation and personal questions should be avoided
- Questions should be pretested
- Instructions, consent, purpose, foot note, whereever necessary are added

(b) Secondary data: The data are collected by the other person but utilized by the investigator for his use. The source is known as records.

Records: They are maintained in registers or books over a long period of time for various purposes. They are mainly used in retrospective type of studies. They also provide trends in the community about health and disease.

Other important sources of data are Govt. publications like five year plans, census data, economic survey, NFHS, NSSO, annual budgets, WHO publications and other semi govternment publications.

Table 12.3: Difference between primary and secondary data

Primary data	Secondary data
Those data, which were collected for the first time	Those data, which have already been collected by some other person
Original in nature and having first hand information	Not original
These are like raw material to which statistical methods are applied	These are like finished products as they have already been statistically applied.
These have been collected for a definite purpose	They are used for the purpose of reviewer of some writing

METHODS OF COLLECTING DATA

There are two main ways for statistical enquiry
1. Census methods (complete enumeration survey)
2. Sampling method
Before this, let us understand two terms:

Universe: It is the aggregate of a specified group of similar objects or individuals, e.g. village, city or country can be represented as a specified group. Total patients suffering from a disease are also an example of population. Children in the age group of 0–5 years or women in the age of 15–45 years are examples of population.

Sample: A part of statistical population selected according to some rule or plan for drawing conclusion regarding the population is called a sample. It is true representative of population and free from bias.

1. **Census method:** In this case data is collected for each and every unit of investigation. So this method is also called method of complete enumeration.

    Merits: It is an extensive study, it is free from sample error and there is high degree of accuracy.

    Demerits: it is expensive, needs many investigators and not possible under special circumstances.

2. **Sampling method:** In this method, a part of the universe (instead of every unit of the universe) is studied and on the basis of this part of study, conclusions are drawn for the whole universe.

REQUIREMENTS OF GOOD SAMPLE

- A good sample should be representative of the universe, i.e. it should be chosen at random and the size of the sample should be as large as possible.

- It also depends upon the method of sampling used as it is stated by one of the statician; mere size, of course, does not assure representation, in a sample. A small or stratified sample is apt to be much superior to a large but badly collected sample.
- It should test for accuracy by taking another sample from the universe.

Merits: It is economical, scientific, reliable, simple and quick.

Demerits: The high degree of accuracy is not possible; there is chance of sampling error. This method needs expert. The size of sample and size of universe are also important.

SAMPLING TECHNIQUES

1. **Simple Random Sampling:** It is a method of selecting a sample, so that every possible unit of population has got the same chance of being selected. It is done by draw of lots or by Tipits no.
2. **Systematic Sampling:** When sampling units are given not in a random way but are arranged in a systematic order, by making sampling units systematically at equally spaced intervals in that order. The sample thus obtained is called systematic sample and the method systematic sampling, e.g. if the universe consists of 100 people and we need to study 10 subjects then after arranging them in a order, every nth person will be studied, i.e. 1,11,21…or 5,15,25… where sample is selected by definite system.
3. **Stratified Sampling:** In stratified sampling the whole population is divided into number of homogenous sub-population. This sub-population is called strata. After dividing the population into different strata, sample is drawn from each stratum. This procedure of sampling is called a stratified random sampling. Stratified in the population is done when it is known that the population is heterogeneous. This technique gives more representative sample then the random techniques.
4. **Multistage Sampling:** Suppose we are interested in getting information for the epidemic of measles in Punjab. For the purpose of our study, the districts are first stage unit, village is second stage and household the third stage and then to take sample of human beings would have been fourth stage sampling and so on. Hence, sampling of stages of more than two is called multistage sampling.
5. **Multiphase Sampling:** In this, information is collected from the whole sample and part from the sub samples. These sub samples become smaller and smaller, e.g. in tuberculosis survey, in the first phase mantoux test is done. In the second phase all mantoux positive cases are subjected to sputum examination. In the third phase all the mantoux positive and sputum negative cases are subjected to X- rays. By this technique we can be more purposeful, less laborious and will also be more cost effective.
6. **Cluster Sampling:** In this method, units of population are considered as clusters. For example, mohalla, school, ward, village, town, etc. after selection of cluster, the entire population is studied. The number of cluster and the population to be studied from each cluster will depend upon the aims and objectives. For example, to study the vaccination coverage 30 cluster are selected depending upon the sampling interval (total population divided by 30). From each cluster 7 children are studied. Thus, a sample size of 210 children gives a reasonably good idea about vaccination coverage.
7. **Purposive Sampling:** In purposive sampling, sample units are chosen deliberately to serve a particular purpose.

CLASSIFICATION OF DATA

Classification: It is method of condensing the information. In this process the collected data is stored or arranged into groups and classes according to their nature or similarities.

Types: It is of two types:

A. According to attribute   B. According to class interval

A. According to Attribute

It is used for qualitative data. This is done by two ways:

a. Simple classification

b. Manifold classification

a. Simple classification: We divide the sample/population into two groups and only one attribute is studied.

Table 12.4: Simple classification of data

Attacked	Not attacked	Total
80	20	100

b. Manifold classification (Multiple classifications)

The data is divided into more than two classes, which may be divided into subclasses, and more than one attributes are studied, e.g. attack rate of viral hepatitis according to sex and marital status.

Table 12.5: Manifold classification of data

Sex	Attacked		Not attacked		Total
	Married	Unmarried	Married	Unmarried	
Male	20	32	3	9	64
Female	10	18	3	5	36
Total	30	50	6	14	100

B. According to Class Interval

This classification is applicable to quantitative data, i.e. height, weight, blood pressure, pulse rate, hemoglobin, serum cholesterol.

Characteristic such as hemoglobin varies from person to person. Suppose 100 women are tested for haemoglobin. The list of 100 women's level of hemoglobin is of no value itself. A simple first step towards organizing the data is to list all the possible values between highest and the lowest in order, recording the frequency (*f*) with which each score occurs. This forms a frequency distribution.

Table 12.6: Simple classes of one characterstic (Hb)

Level of Hb	Frequency (f)	
6	9	
7	11	
8	15	If lowest hemoglobin level is 6 and highest level is 14 then this can be a frequency distribution
9	23	
10	13	
11	10	
12	8	
13	6	
14	5	

Grouped frequency distribution: The above data can be made more manageable by creating a grouped frequency distribution. Individual scores are grouped as:

Table 12.7: Class interval with frequency

Hb level with Interval	f	Relative f	Cumulative f
6 – 8	35	35%	100
9 – 11	46	46%	65.0
12 – 14	19	19%	19.0

The data, so collected is divided into a number of classes and these classes are known as class intervals. Here in this case there are three class intervals.

The limit within which a class interval lies is called *class limit*. Here 6 to 8 gm percent is a class limit. 6 gm is lower class limit and 8 gm is the upper class limit.

The difference between the upper and lower class limits of a *class interval* is called class magnitude. Here 2 gm is magnitude, i.e. 6 to 8 gm (8 – 6 = 2 gm).

The number of persons present in one class interval is known as class frequency.

POINTS TO REMEMBER

1. The class interval should be determined in accordance with the size of the data.
2. The class interval should be preferably of uniform magnitude.
3. Class limits should be so fixed in a manner to display the main characteristics of the distribution accurately.
4. The class limit should be preferably a whole number.
5. The grouped data should not look very small or very large.
6. Intermediate classes may be avoided.

13

Presentation of Data

METHODS OF PRESENTATION OF DATA

There are two main methods: (I) Tabulation (II) Diagrams

Principles of Presentation

1. To arrange the data in such a way that it elevates interest in a reader.
2. To make the data sufficiently precise, without loosing important details.
3. The presentation of data should be done in a way that it shows pattern of variation clearly.
4. To present the data in a simple form in order to make it possible to form some impressions and draw some conclusions directly or indirectly.
5. To help in further statistical analysis.

I. Tabulation

It is the presentation of classified data in a systematic and scientific way and in form, so that special features of the data are clear.

Guidelines for Tabulation

i. Table drawn should be attractive, impressive and clear.
ii. Due prominence should be given to title and subtitle.
iii. The title should be clear, simple and should give complete description.
iv. Data must be presented according to size or albhabetically.
v. The rows and columns should be serialized and heading should be clear and concise.
vi. The unit of measurement should be specified and defined.
vii. Full details of deliberate exclusion of observations in a collected series must be given.
viii. Complicated tables should be avoided.
ix. A table should be self-explanatory.
x. It should be easily read and understood, so that there is no wastage of time.
xi. The source of material should be mentioned clearly.
xii. Footnotes should be written wherever essential.

Table 13.1: Distribution of patients according to speciality in 2008*

	Speciality	Number of patients
1.	Oral medicine and radiology	315
2.	Oral surgery	280
3.	Pedodontics	105
4.	Orthodontics	85
5.	Conservative dentistry and endodontics	235
	Total	**1086**

*Source: Central registration, GDC, Amritsar

Frequency Distribution Tables

Here the data is first split up into convenient groups, i.e. class intervals and number of items, i.e. frequency that occurs in each group is shown in Table 13.2.

Table 13.2: Data with class interval and frequency

Age in years	Number of persons suffering from Caries
0 – 5	2
5 – 10	5
10 – 15	10
15 – 20	15
20 – 25	3
25 – 30	4

Remember: The aim of a biostatistician is different from a statistician or person with pure mathematical background. It is true that the class interval should be equal and precise. However, look at this distribution table:

Age group

0 – 1

1 – 5

5 – 15

16 – 45

45 – 65

> 65

Of course, it looks odd from the statistical norm, but it is more informative as the first group is of infancy, 1–5 years are preschool years, 5–15 are school going children, 16–45 is reproductive age group, 45 to 65 is middle age and more than 65 is old age or geriatric group. We can conclude according to their specific problems. Similarly adolescent age is 10 to 19 years, it is further divided into pre adolescent, middle adolescent and late adolescent. So, the knowledge of medical science and the area of thrust must be kept in mind while applying the rules of statistics and should be altered keeping in view the inferences we want to draw.

II. Diagrams

These are meant for non-statistical minded people and general public, who need only an impression of the relative value of frequencies of persons and events.

- These are methods or aids, which facilitate understanding of data.
- They are a good method for comparison.

The fundamental problem of diagrammatic presentation is to select the most appropriate method, out of various alternatives available for making comparison. The success of choices made, lies in the speed and accuracy with which the comparison is made for understanding the figures.

The diagrammatic presentation will depend upon the type of data and purposes for which it is required.

Table 13.3: Relationship between type of data and type of diagram

Type of data	Type of diagram
Qualitative/Discrete	Bar diagram, pie diagram, pictogram, spot maps
Quantitative/Continuous	Histogram, Frequency polygon, Frequency curve, Line chart, Cumulative frequency diagram, Scatter or dot diagram

PRESENTATION OF QUALITATIVE DATA

Bar Diagram

- It is a method of diagrammatic presentation of frequency data (discrete data).
- The length of the bar is proportional to class frequencies.
- These give visual impression for comparison of the magnitude of different frequencies in discrete data.

The bars can be vertical, horizontal, and multiple or comprise of various components depending upon the type of data and purpose of analysis.

Pie or Sector Diagram

- This is another way of presenting discrete data of qualitative character in which a circle is divided into various sectors.

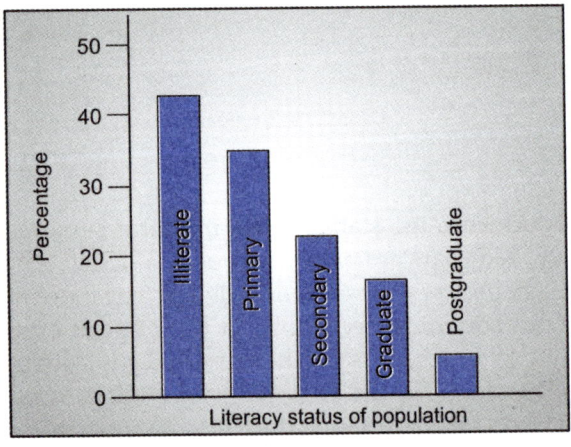

Fig. 13.1: Bar diagram showing literacy status of Punjab

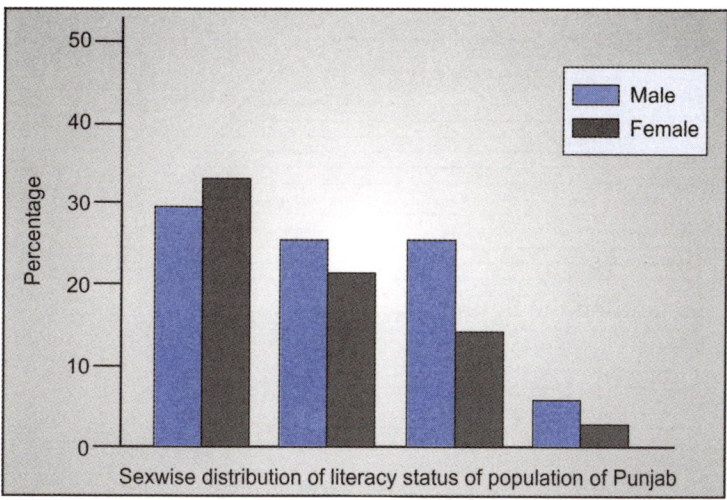

Fig. 13.2: Multiple bar diagram showing sexwise distribution of literacy status of Punjab

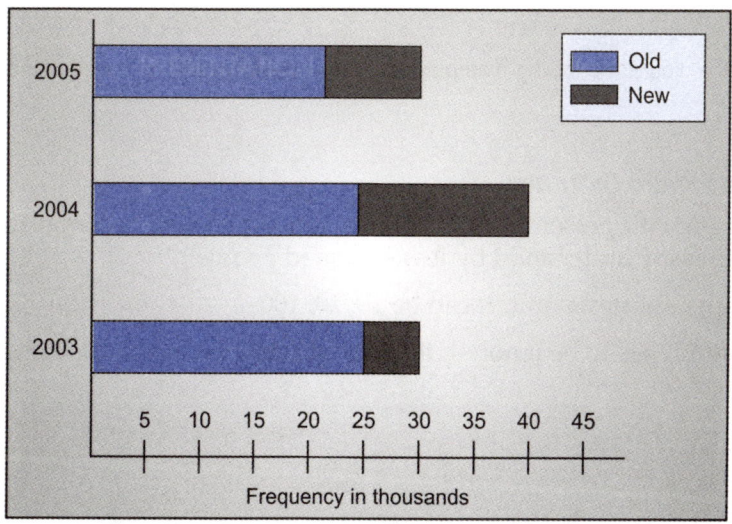

Fig. 13.3: Components of bar diagram showing cases of cervical abrasions

- Degree of angles and area of sectors are proportional to the class frequencies.
- The area of the sectors is usually given in percentage.

Example: 200 persons distributed according to socio-economic status

Table 13.4: Cases according to socio-economic status

Socio-economic status	Cases	% age	Degree presentation
Class I	20	10	$20 \times 360/200 = 36°$
Class II	40	20	$40 \times 360/200 = 72°$
Class III	100	50	$100 \times 360/200 = 180°$
Class IV	40	20	$40 \times 360/200 = 72°$

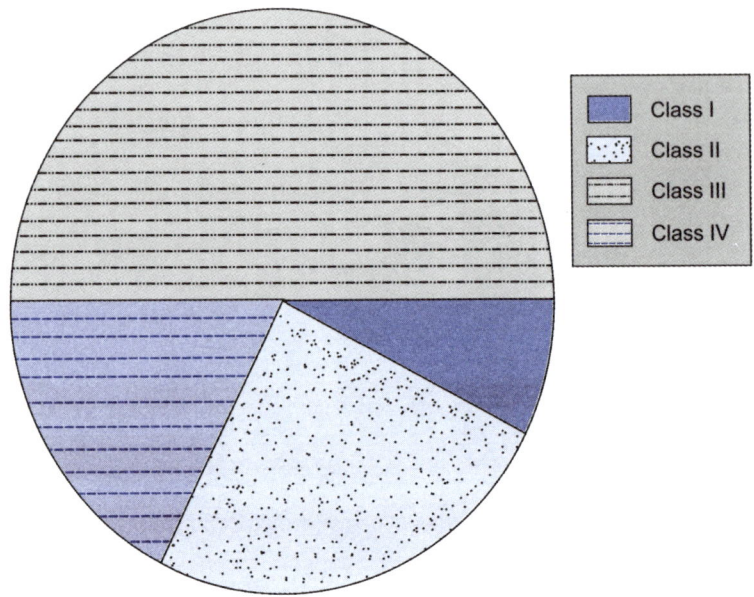

▨	Class I
⋯	Class II
☰	Class III
☰	Class IV

Fig. 13.4: Pie diagram showing distribution of persons according to socio-economic status

Pictogram or Picture Diagram

- It is a diagrammatic presentation in which pictures or symbols denote the frequency. This can be easily understood by less educated people.
- Each picture indicates a unit. It can be 10, 20, 100
- Fraction of unit has to be ignored, though half may be indicated by half a picture.

Village	Cases	Each figure representing 10
A	40	𝆘 𝆘 𝆘 𝆘
B	50	𝆘 𝆘 𝆘 𝆘 𝆘
C	25	𝆘 𝆘 𝆘

Fig. 13.5: Pictogram showing cases of dental caries in three villages

Spot Maps or Map Diagram

These are mostly used for depicting frequencies or number of persons having or suffering from a disease in defined geographical areas.

These are shaded with different colours for easy differentiation.

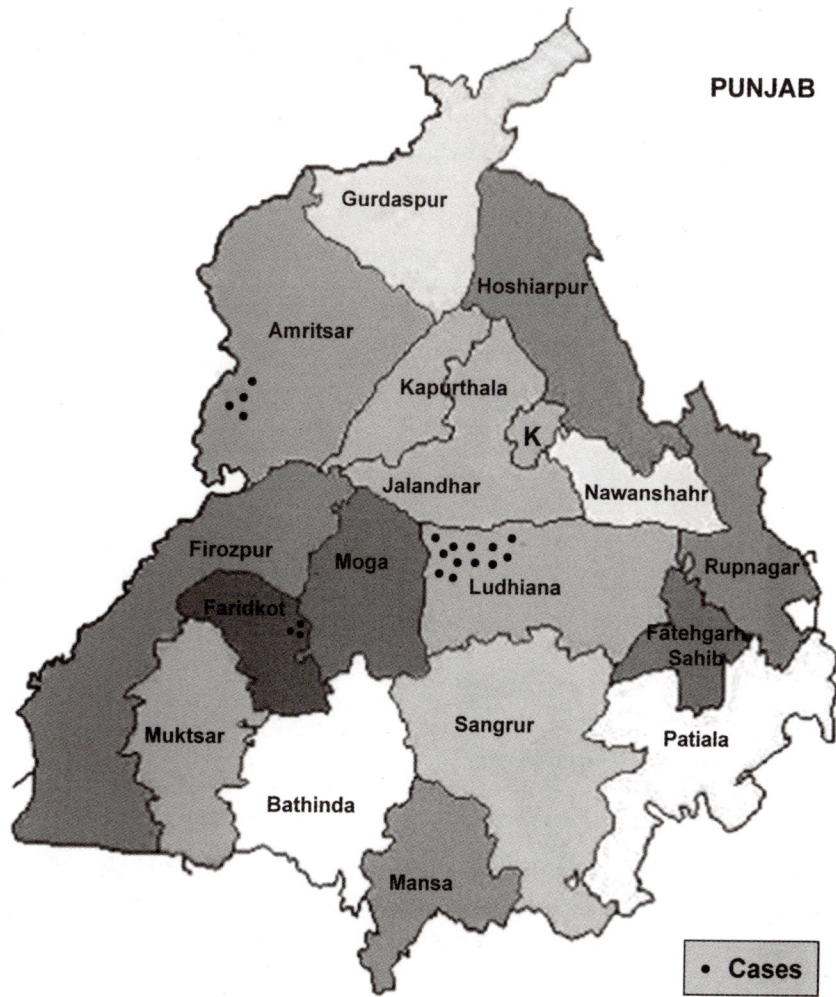

Fig. 13.6: Spot map showing cases of polio in 2009

PRESENTATION OF QUANTITATIVE DATA

Histogram

It is the graphical presentation of frequency distribution of quantitative or continuous data.
The independent variable is plotted along the base and the frequencies along the vertical axis.

Table 13.5: Frequency distribution of grouped data

Interval	Frequency (f)	Relative frequency (%)	Cumulative frequency (%)
161 – 170	4	2.0	2.0
171 – 180	5	2.5	4.5
181 – 190	12	6.0	10.5
191 – 200	14	7.0	17.5

Table 13.5: Frequency distribution of grouped data (*Contd.*)

Interval	Frequency (f)	Relative frequency (%)	Cumulative frequency (%)
201 – 210	72	36.0	53.5
211 – 220	38	19.0	72.5
221 – 230	18	9.0	81.5
231 – 240	19	9.5	91.0
241 – 250	13	6.5	97.5
251 – 260	5	2.5	100.0

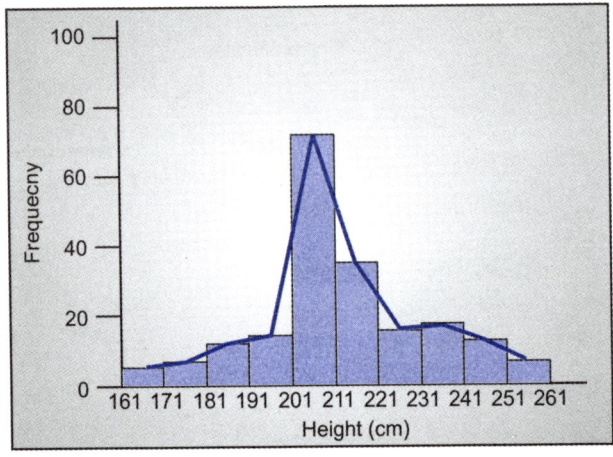

Fig. 13.7: Histogram showing height of students of a class

- Frequency of each group will form a column or rectangle. It is also known as Area Diagram, as area of the rectangle is proportional to class frequency.
- The height of rectangle alone will indicate the frequency, if the class interval is uniform.

Frequency Polygon

It is a diagrammatic presentation of frequency distribution with class frequencies plotted against class mid point and the points being joined by straight lines.

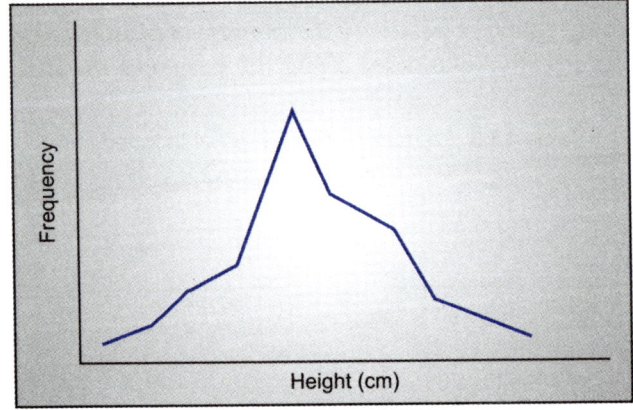

Fig. 13.8: Frequency polygon showing height of students of a class

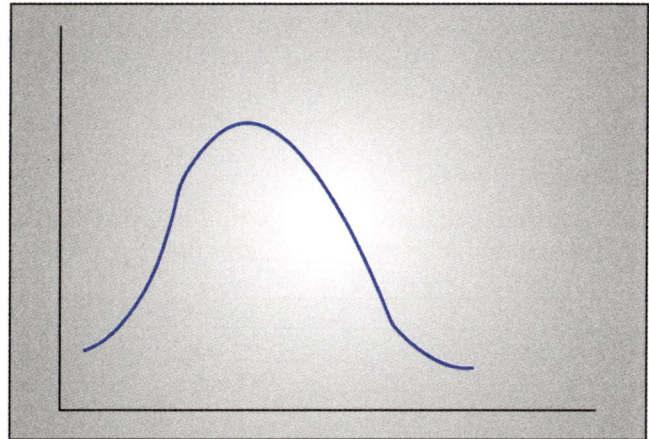

Fig. 13.9: Frequency curve showing distribution of data

This can also be obtained by joining mid points of the rectangles of a histogram.

Frequency Curve

When the number of observations is very large and group interval is reduced, the frequency polygon tends to lose its angulations, giving place to a smooth curve known as frequency curve. This provides continuous graph as seen in normal distributive curve.

Ogive or Cumulative Frequency Diagram

It can be presented graphically as a polygon. It forms a characteristic S-shaped curve known as ogive.

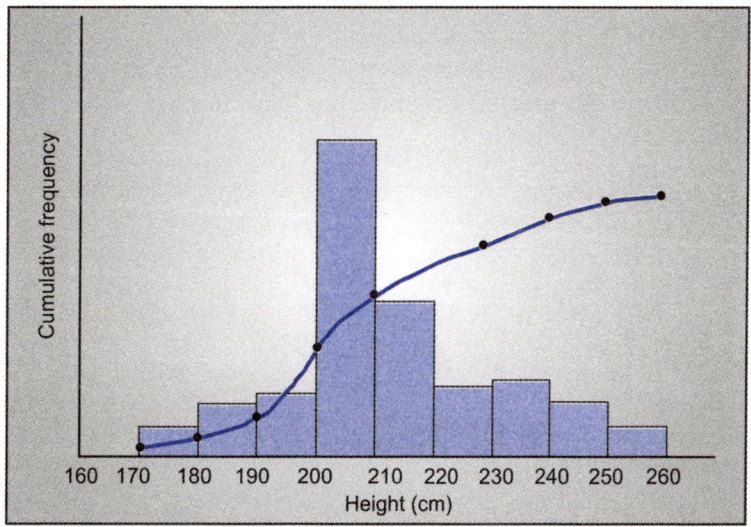

Fig. 13.10: Ogive or cumulative frequency diagram showing height of students of a class

From this, we can locate percentiles, i.e. states the percentage of observations that fall below any particular score or one can say centile ranks states that percentage of observations that fall within or below any given class interval. It provides a way of giving information about one individual score in relation to all the other scores in a distribution.

For example, in the above diagram 91% observations fall below 240.5 mg/lt. The figure of 240.5 mg/lt, therefore represents the 91st centile, which means approximately 9% of the scores in the sample are higher than this value or this person. A person can be told about his value that how much is his rank in the population.

Line Chart or Line Graph

It shows the trend of an event occurring over a period of time (whether event is rising, falling or showing fluctuation, i.e. birth rate, death rate or population, etc).

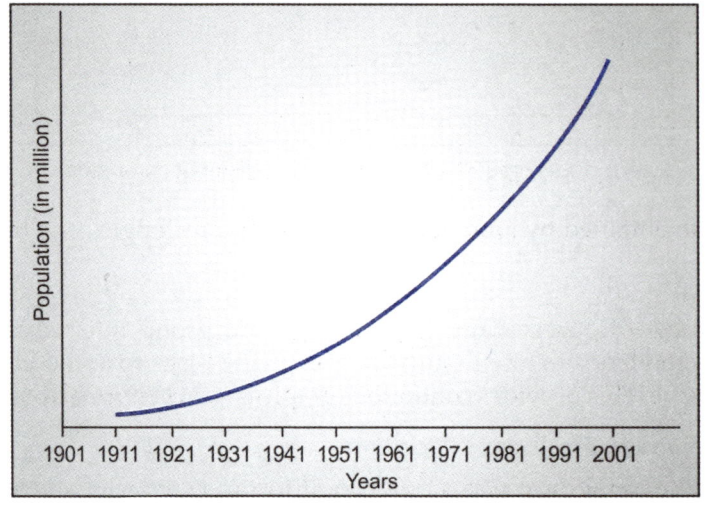

Fig. 13.11: Line diagram showing population trend from 1901 to 2001

Scatter or Dot Diagram

It is drawn to show nature of correlation between two variables, e.g. height (X) and weight (Y) in persons or groups of the same age. The characters are read on base line (height) and vertical (weight) axis.

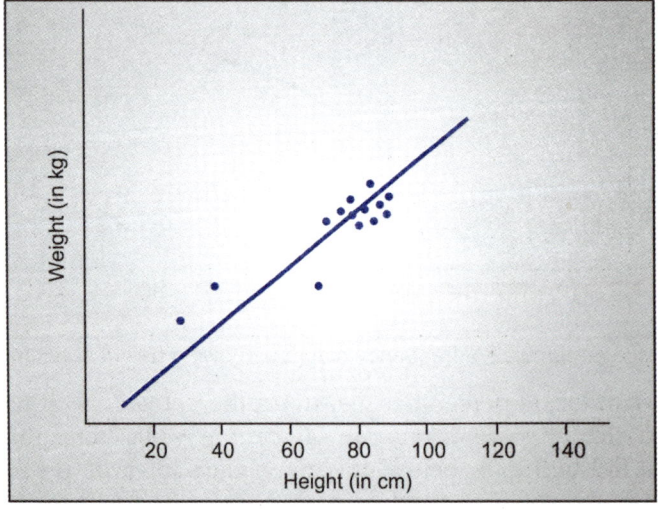

Fig. 13.12: Scatter diagram showing height of students of a class

14

Analysis of Data

We have learnt about the methods of collection and presentation of data. Now, we have to understand and grasp the application of mathematical techniques involved in analysis and interpretation of data.

Researchers usually characterize an entire distribution by one typical figure that represents all the observations. Such figures are:

  I. Measure of central tendency, i.e. average
 II. Measure of locations, i.e. percentiles
III. Measure of dispersion, i.e variability

MEASURE OF CENTRAL TENDENCY

In any data, there exists a tendency to cluster (gather) around the central value, i.e. central tendency. This describes the center of the group and divides the distribution approximately in two equal parts. In any large series, nearly 50% observations lie above while the remaining 50% lies below the central value. It indicates how the values lie near the center. Thus, an average value helps us in the following manner:

i. Most common observations lie close to central value while few which are too large or too small, lie away at both ends.

ii. For comparing the averages of one group with that of another. So, on finding a difference one may reason out why in one group it is more than in the other. The average height of women is more in Punjab as compared to Tamil Nadu or per capita income of Punjab is more.

There are three measures of central tendency in common use, i.e. Mean, Median and Mode.

Mean (Arithmetic average): It is the sum of all the observations divided by the number of elements in the distribution.

$$\text{Mean} = \frac{\text{Sum of all the observations}}{\text{Total number of observations}}$$

or

$$= \frac{x_1 + x_2 + x_3 + \dots + x_n}{n}$$

- Mean responds to the exact value of every observation in the distribution.
- It is very sensitive to extreme values.
- It is not usually an appropriate measure for characterizing very skewed distributions.

Calculation of mean in different type of series is as:

A. Ungrouped data

   a. For small number of observations, e.g.

     B.P. of ten individuals is

     83, 75, 81, 79, 71, 75, 95, 77, 84, 90

       i. Add all

      ii. Divide by total number of observations

$$\text{Mean} = \frac{83 + 75 + 81 + 79 + 71 + 95 + 77 + 84 + 90}{10} = \frac{810}{10} = 81$$

   b. For large number of observations

       i. Assume an arbitrary mean

      ii. Find out the difference between each measurement and assumed mean

     iii. Sum up differences

     iv. Divide by total number of observations

      v. Calculate original mean by:

Mean = Assumed mean + Mean of differences, e.g. 10 persons having B.P. Take assumed mean as 80.

Table 14.1: Calculation of mean in an ungrouped data

Obs.	Assured mean	difference from mean
84	80	− 4
75	80	− 5
80	80	0
79	80	+ 1
71	80	+ 9
75	80	+ 5
95	80	− 15
77	80	+ 3
84	80	− 4
90	80	− 10
Total		**− 20**

    Sum of difference = − 20

$$\text{After dividing} = \frac{-20}{10} = -2$$

$$\text{Mean} = 80 + (-2)$$
$$= 80 - 2$$
$$= 78$$

B. Grouped series, i.e. for frequency distribution table when observations are large in number (Table 14.2).

   a. For discrete series

       i. Take product of frequency and value of observations

      ii. Divide by total number of observations (frequency)

Table 14.2: Calculation of mean in descrete series

Days of hospital stay	Number of patients	Total days of each group
6	5	30
7	4	28
8	4	32
9	3	27
10	2	20
	18	**137**

$$\therefore \quad \text{Mean} = 137/18 = 7.61$$

b. For continuous series (Table 14.3)

   i. Take mid value of class interval

   ii. Take product of mid value with frequency

   iii. Divide by total number of observations

Table 14.3: Calculation of mean in continuous series

Age in years	Frequency	Mid value	Product
11 – 13	3	12	36
13 – 15	4	14	56
15 – 17	5	16	80
17 – 19	6	18	108
19 – 21	5	20	100
21 – 23	4	22	88
23 – 25	3	24	72
	30		**540**

$$\therefore \quad \text{Mean} = 540/30 = 18$$

Merits

- Simple to calculate
- No need for arranging the data
- Easy to understand
- Useful for further statistical analysis

Demerits

- It is calculated from all the observations, thus if there are very big or small observations in the series, it will give abnormal result.
- Values of all the items are necessary for calculating mean.
- Sometimes the mean cannot be a figure, which does not exist in the observations, e.g. six children having number of teeth erupted at 2 years are: 3, 5, 8, 9, 7, 4 and mean of all is 6, which is not present in any of the child.
- Sometime it gives absurd results as 2.3 children per family.

Median: It is the value of the middle item of a series when data is arranged in ascending or descending order of magnitude. It divides a series into two equal halves. In one half, the values are less than the median and in the other half, more than the median.

When a distribution has an odd number of elements, the median is the middle one; when it has an even number of elements, the median lies halfway between the two middle scores, e.g. in a distribution consisting of elements 6, 9, 15, 17, 24, the median would be 15, but if the distributions were 6, 9, 15, 17, 24, 29, the median would be 16 (average of 15 and 17).

Note that median responds only to the number of scores above and below it, not to their values. The median is a better indicator of the central value as it is insensitive to small number of extreme scores in a distribution.

For example, Absenteeism of school children in the series are:

4, 6, 8, 10, 12, 14, 37

Median = 10

Mean = 91/7 = 13

In this case, mean value gives a wrong idea, as the observation 37 is too large.

If one large observation is ignored then:

54/6 = 9 is mean, which is much closer to median (10) as compared to mean of series, i.e. 13.

Median = value in the arranged series, where n is number of observations, which is an odd number.

For example, 83, 75, 81, 79, 71, 95, 75, 77, 84

Arrange series: 71, 75, 75, 77, 79, 81, 83, 84, 95

$$\text{Median} = \left(\frac{n+1}{2}\right)^{th} = \left(\frac{9+1}{2}\right)^{th} = \text{5th value, i.e. 79.}$$

For grouped series (Table 14.4):

$$\text{Median} = l + \frac{(n/2 - f)^c}{x}$$

l = lower limit of median group

n = total number of observations

f = Total number of observations up to median group

c = class width of median group

x = Total number of observations in the median group

Table 14.4: Calculation of median in grouped series

Age groups	Number of patients	Cumulative frequency
0 – 10	46	46
11 – 20	66	112
21 – 30	56	168
31 – 40	88	256
41 – 50	101	357
51 – 60	68	425
61 – 70	25	450

Median group = 31 – 40

l = 31

n = 450

$$f = 168$$
$$c = 10$$
$$x = 88$$

$$\text{Median} = l + \frac{(n/2 - f)^c}{x} = 31 + \frac{(450/2 - 168)^{10}}{88} = 37.4$$

Merits of Median

- Easy to calculate
- Understood without difficulty
- Not effected by the values of extreme items and can be calculated, if the number of observations is known.
- Sometimes more representative than mean.

Demerits

- It is not representative of series in many cases. This is specially so, when there are wide variations between the values of different items and the sample size is small.
- Arrangement of data is time consuming and tedious.

Mode: It is the most frequently occurring observation in the series, i.e. the most common or fashionable item.

It is determined by simple inspection of the frequency distribution. If two scores occur with the greater frequency, the distribution is bimodal. Sometimes it can be multimodal due to more than two values occurring frequently in the series.

It is also uninfluenced by the small number of extreme values in the distribution.

For example, Protein content of various varieties of wheat is as under:

11, 8, 8, 9, 10, 11, 12, 8, 9, 11

Mode in this is 11, or bimodal value 11 and 8.

For grouped series: The formula is:

$$\text{Mode} = l_m + \frac{f_1 c}{f_1 + f_2}$$

l_m = lower limit of modal group

f_1 = total number of observations in a modal group minus total number of observations in the group preceding the modal group

f_2 = total number of observations in a modal group minus total number of observations in the group following the modal group

c = class width of modal group

If we want to calculate 'Mode' from the data given in Table 14.4, then steps are:

Modal group = 41 – 50, l_m = 41, f_1 = 101–88, f_2 = 101 – 68, c = 10

$$\text{Mode} = l_m + \frac{f_1 c}{f_1 + f_2} = 41 + \frac{13 \times 10}{13 + 33} = 41 + \frac{130}{46} = 43.8$$

RELATIONSHIP BETWEEN MEAN, MEDIAN AND MODE

The relationship of the three measures depends upon the shape of distribution.

In unimodal symmetrical distribution, i.e. in normal distribution it is identical, i.e. Mean = Median = Mode.

But in general, they differ in skewed distributions, which can be positively skewed or negatively skewed.

In both the cases, mode is simply the most frequently occurring value. The mean is influenced by relatively small number of very high and very low scores and the median lies between the two, dividing the distributions into two equal halves.

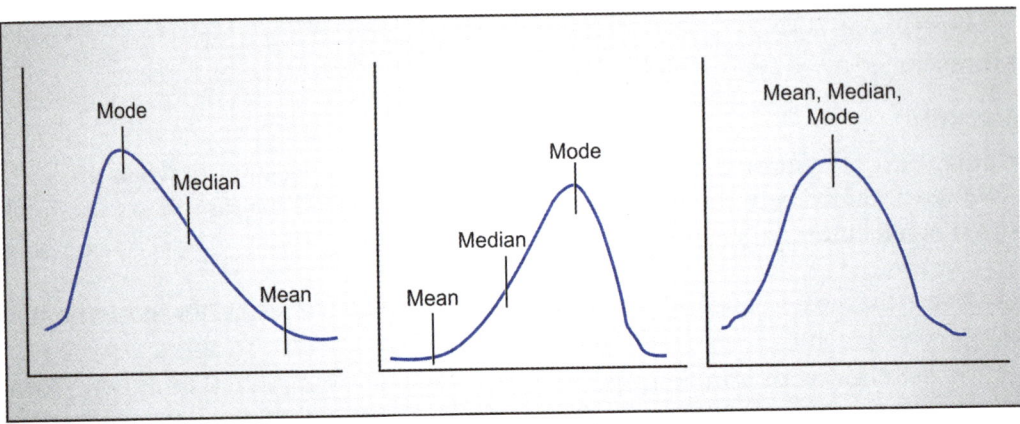

Fig. 14.1: Frequency curves in relation to various types of data with difference of mean, mode and median

WHEN TO USE THE MEASURES OF CENTRAL TENDENCY

Mean

1. When the number (scores) is (are) distributed symmetrically around a central point, i.e. more or less the normal distribution.
2. When greater stability is wanted.s
3. When the measures like standard deviation, coefficient of correlation are to be computed later.

Median

1. When exact mid point of distribution is wanted, i.e. 50% point.
2. When there are extreme points, which are going to affect the mean.

Mode

1. When quick and approximate measures of central tendency is all that wanted.
2. When the measure of central tendency should be the most typical value.

15

Measures of Location–Percentiles

Averages discussed so for are measures of central value, therefore they locate at the centre or midpoint of a distribution. It may be of interest to locate other points in the range. Percentiles do that. Thus, percentiles or partition values divide the series into more than two parts. Those commonly used are:

1. Median
2. Quartiles
3. Quintiles
4. Deciles
5. Percentiles

Median: It divides the whole series of observations into two equal parts; each part will have 50% of the total observations on each side of median.

Quartiles: There are three quartiles in a series—Q_1, Q_2, and Q_3. it divides the series into 4 equal parts. Each part has 25% observations of a series falling on its left and 75% on its right.

Quintiles: They are four in numbers (Quin-1, Quin-2, Quin-3, Quin-4) and divide the series into 5 equal parts, each having 20% of total observation. So, first quintile will have 20% observations falling to its left and 80% to its right.

Deciles: They are 9 in number (D_1, D_2, ..., D_9) and divide the series in 10 equal parts. Each decile is 10% of total observations.

Percentiles: They are 99 in number (P_1, P_2, ..., P_{99}) and divide the series in 100 equal parts. Each percentile having 1% observations.

Thus,   Median $= Q_2 = D_5 = P_{50}$
$$Q_1 = P_{25}$$

CALCULATION OF PERCENTILES

$$\text{Median} = \text{the size of } \left(\frac{n+1}{2}\right)^{\text{th}} \text{ term}$$

$$Q_1 = \text{the size of } \left(\frac{n+1}{4}\right)^{\text{th}} \text{ term}$$

$$Q_3 = \text{the size of } 3\left(\frac{n+1}{4}\right)^{th} \text{ term}$$

$$Quin_1 = \text{the size of }\left(\frac{n+1}{5}\right)^{th} \text{ term}$$

$$Quin_2 = \text{the size of } 2\left(\frac{n+1}{5}\right)^{th} \text{ term}$$

$$D_1 = \text{the size of }\left(\frac{n+1}{10}\right)^{th} \text{ term}$$

$$D_6 = \text{the size of } 6\left(\frac{n+1}{10}\right)^{th} \text{ term}$$

$$P_1 = \text{the size of }\left(\frac{n+1}{100}\right)^{th} \text{ term}$$

$$P_{99} = \text{the size of } 99\left(\frac{n+1}{100}\right)^{th} \text{ term}$$

Ungrouped Series

Diastolic blood pressure of 10 subjects is:

1	2	3	4	5	6	7	8	9	10
71	75	76	77	79	81	83	84	90	95

Median= $(n +1)/2$ or $(10 +1)/2 = 5.5$, observation against serial number 5 is 79.

So, $79 + 0.5 (81 - 79)$ or $79+ 0.5 \times 2 = 80$

$Q_1 = (n + 1)/4$ or $(10 + 1)/4 = 2.75$ $75 + 0.75 (76 - 75) = 75.75$

$Q_3 = 3 (n + 1)/4$ or $3(10 +1)/4 = 8.25$ $84 + 0.25 (90 - 84) = 85.50$

Grouped Series

- To find the percentiles in grouped series, simply divide the total observation by 2. If total is 200, 100th observation is the mid value. Even if the total is 201, the 100th observation may be taken as mid value or median.
- The Median, Quartile, Quintile, Decile and Percentile value of the characteristics can be calculated from the cumulative frequency table. Find the variable group in which the particular value lies.
- Then raise the lower value of the variable of that group proportionately to the value of that particular observation with the presumption that rises from lower value to the higher value is uniform.

Alternate Method

Percentiles $= l_1 + (l_2 - l_1)/f_1 \times (p - c)$ $p = n/100$

$l_1 = $ lower limit of class interval in which percentile lies

$l_2 = $ Upper limit of class interval in which percentile lies

$f_1 = $ Frequency of class interval in which percentile lies

p = Middle line of class interval in which percentile lies

c = Cumulative frequency preceding to class interval in which percentile lies.

Median = $l_1 + (l_2 - l_1)/f_1 \times (m - c)$ $m = n/2$

$Q_1 = l_1 + (l_2 - l_1)/f_1 \times (q_1 - c)$ $q_1 = n/4$

$Q_3 = l_1 + (l_2 - l_1)/f_1 \times (q_3 - c)$ $q_3 = (3 \times n)/4$

$D_6 = l_1 + (l_2 - l_1)/f_1 \times (d_6 - c)$ $d_6 = (6 \times n)/10$

$P_{55} = l_1 + (l_2 - l_1)/f_1 \times (p_{55} - c)$ $p_{55} = (55 \times n)/100$

Table 15.1: Cumulative frequency

Height in cm.	Frequency	Cumulative frequency
160–162	10	10
162–164	15	25
164–166	17	42
166–168	19	61
168–170	20	81
170–172	26	107
172–174	29	136
174–176	30	166
176-178	22	188
178–180	12	200

Median = Quartile 2 = Deciles 5 = Percentiles 50

Median, i.e. 200/2 or 100th observation lies in the height group 170–172 cm.

81 is the cumulative frequency up to 170 cm.

The frequency rises by 19 from 81to 100 (i.e. middle observation).

For 26 observations (81–107), the attribute value rises by 2 cm from 170–172.

Therefore, proportionate rise in attribute will be:

$$2 \times (100 - 81)/26 = (2 \times 19)/26 = 1.46$$

Thus,   Median = 170 + 1.46 = 171.46 cm

MEASUREMENT OF VARIABILITY

Although measures of central tendency are very useful to summarize a frequency distribution but they do not indicate the spread of values around the average.

We can take this example (Table 15.2).

Table 15.2: Variability of various types

Sr. No.	Temperature observed	Mean
1	0 – 100°C	50
2	40 – 60°C	50
3	49 – 51°C	50

Here mean is same in all the conditions but it does not convey any idea about the distribution of the individual values.

Again we can understand it from normal distribution.

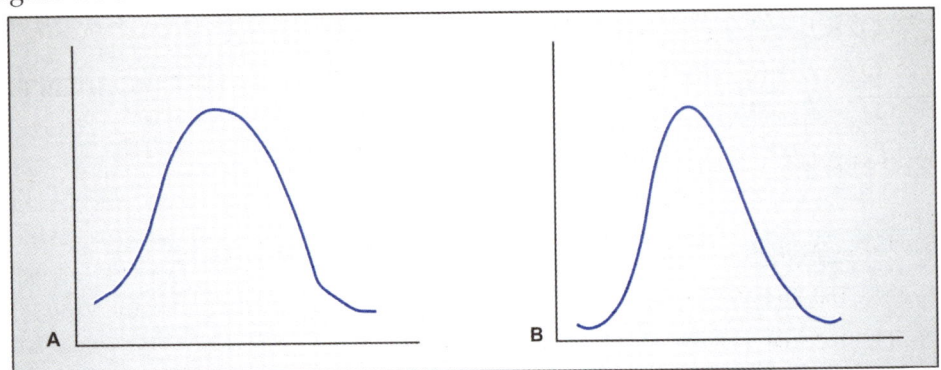

Fig. 15.1: Various types of normal distribution

These two norml distribution curves are similar. Mean, Median, Mode are equal in these two curves as they are symmetrical and bell shaped. Despite their similarities, these two distributions are different. So, these measures are not adequate.

These two examples show that there is a difference of distribution in terms of their variability.

The values distributed in Fig. 15.1(A) are more scattered as compared to Fig. 15.1(B).

If these two distributions are representing the fasting blood sugar of two different hypoglycemic agents then drug B would be better medication, as fewer patients on the distribution have very high or very low blood sugar, even though the mean effect of drug B is the same as that of drug A.

The important measures of variability are:

  i. Range

 ii. Mean deviation

iii. Variance

iv. Standard deviation

i. Range

It is the simplest measure of variability. It measures the scatter of the values of variable. It is the absolute difference between highest and lowest value and ignore the distribution of all the observations in between these values.

- It changes with change in sample
- It is a rough comparison
- The range of symmetrical and asymmetrical distribution can be identical.

From the above table, out of three examples range is 0 – 100, 40 to 60 and 49 to 51 with a different or range of 100, 20 and 2.

ii. Mean Deviation

It is the arithmetic average of the absolute deviations of the values of the observations from mean.

Though it is simple and easy, it is not used in statistical analysis being the only mathematical value.

Calculation of Mean Deviation

1. Calculate the mean of the series.
2. Take deviations of each value from the arithmetic mean.
3. Add up the deviations (ignore + or –ve sign)
4. Divide the result by number of observations.

For example, diastolic BP of 10 individuals is given in Table 15.3.

Table 15.3: Calculation of mean deviation

Value	Mean	Deviation from mean
83	81	+2
75	81	– 6
81	81	0
79	81	– 2
71	81	– 10
95	81	+14
75	81	– 6
77	81	– 4
84	81	+3
90	81	+9
810		56 (giving sign)

Mean deviation = 56/10 = 5.6

iii. Variance

It is the mean of the square of all the deviation scores in the distribution.

Table 15.4: Calculation of variance

Value	Deviation from mean	Square of deviation from mean
83	+ 2	4
75	– 6	36
81	0	0
79	– 2	4
71	– 10	100
95	– 14	196
75	– 6	36
77	– 4	16
84	+ 3	9
90	+ 9	81
Total = 810		Total = 470

Total = 810/10 = 81

= 470/10 = 47

This is not useful most of the time due to its squared units of measurement.

iv. Standard Deviation

It is the square root of the variance, i.e. it is the mean square deviation and the root has been calculated. It is more important than mean deviation and it is expressed in the same units as the original data, so it is used for further statistical analysis as compared to variance.

$$SD = \text{Root mean square deviation}$$

Steps for calculation:

1. Find mean of the series.
2. Take deviation of each value from the arithmetic mean.
3. Take square of each deviation.
4. Add up the squared deviations.
5. Divide the total square of deviation by number of observations (n) or ($n-1$).
6. Take the square root

$$SD = \sqrt{\frac{\Sigma(x - \bar{x})^2}{n-1}} = \sqrt{\text{Variance}}$$

From the data of Table 15.4, $\quad SD = \sqrt{\frac{470}{10-1}} = \sqrt{\frac{470}{9}} = \sqrt{53.3} = 7.28$

Uses of Standard Deviation

1. It summarizes the variation of a large distribution from the mean into one figure and defines limits of variation (normality).
2. It measures the distance of an observation from the central tendency or mean.
3. It helps us to calculate standard error of mean which helps us to find out whether the difference between mean of two different series is by chance or due to some external error.
4. It helps us to determine size of sample for study purpose.
5. It is used for comparing the same character in two different series or two characters in the same series by coefficient of variation.

Limitations of Standard Deviation

1. SD of two quantitative series cannot be compared, if the values pertain to different attributes such as weight and height.
2. Two values, if pertain to the same attribute and have different units of measurement are considered to belong to two different series, i.e. inches and cm cannot be compared.

Coefficient of Variation

Here value of SD is expressed as percentage of the mean.
It is a unit less number, so value may be in any unit, it is well suited for that.

EXERCISES TO SOLVE

1. Average weight of baby at birth is 3.1 kg with standard deviation of 0.4 kg. If the birth weights are normally distributed, would you regard:

    a. weight of 4 kg as normal?

    b. weight of 2.6 kg as normal?

2. Following stillbirth rate 1000 total births were reported by 30 towns in 1977.

    27, 28, 40, 32, 30   36, 25, 29, 30, 29

    36, 37, 29, 29, 42   32, 27, 35, 36,29

            26, 30, 20, 35, 32

            33, 27, 41, 49, 34

    I. Prepare a frequency table and draw a line graph

    II. Calculate mean, median and S.D.

3. Compare variability of SBP in children of age group 5 – 10 years, with that of adults of age group 30–40 years. The data is as follows

Group	Mean	SD
Children	100.8	
Adults	120	12

4. Total serum proteins (in gm percent) of 31 subjects are as under

    7.8, 7.2, 7.0, 6.8, 7.4, 7.2, 7.2, 7.4, 7.2, 6.6, 7.1, 7.3, 7.5, 7.4, 7.4, 7.2, 7.2, 6.6, 7.1, 7.3, 7.5, 7.4, 7.2, 7.2, 6.9, 5.8, 7.2, 7.3, 7.0, 7.3, 6.8

    Determine the range, mean, SD.

16

Normal Distribution and Normal Curve

If large number of observations of any variable are taken at random to make it a representative sample and with a small class interval, a frequency distribution table is prepared then it will be observed that:

1. Some observations are above the mean and others are below the mean.

2. If the observations are arranged in order deviating towards the extreme from mean on plus or minus side, maximum number of frequencies will be seen in the middle around the mean and fewer at the extremes, decreasing smoothly on both the sides.

3. Normally half of the above and half below the mean and all observations are symmetrically distributed on each side of mean.

Table 16.1: Normal distribution of a large sample

Height in cm	Frequency
142.5 – 145 ·	3
145 – 147.5	8
147.5 – 150	15
150 – 155	45
155 – 157.5	155
157.4 – 160	194
160 – 162.5	195
165–167.5	93
167.5–170	42
170 –172.5	16
172.5–175	6
175 – 177.5	2

Mean ± 1 SD = 680 = 68%

Mean ± 2 SD = 950 = 95%

Mean ± 3 SD = 995 = 99.5%

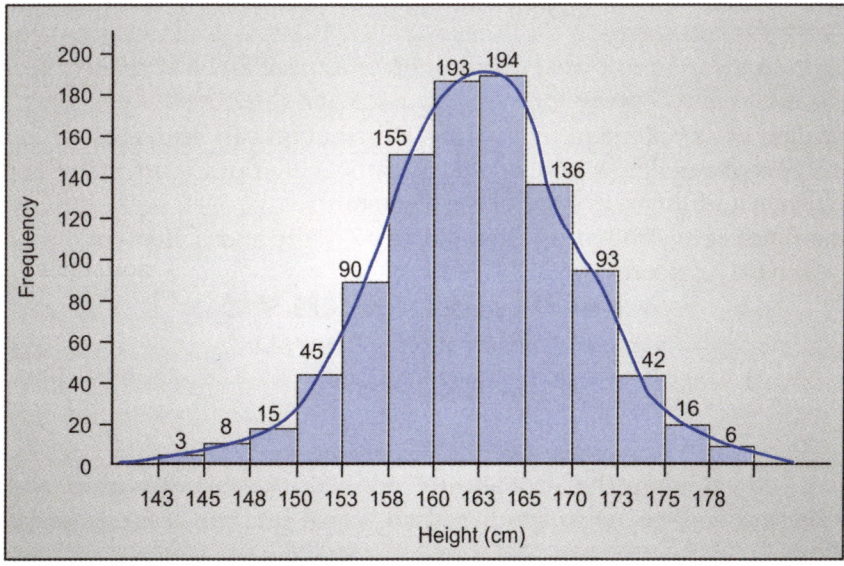

Fig. 16.1: Normal distribution curve

A distribution of this nature is called Normal Distribution. Arithmetically, it can be expressed on term of mean and SD, if they are known:

1. Mean ± 1 SD limits include = 68.2% of total observations
2. Mean ± 2SD limits include = 95.45% of total observations
3. Mean ± 1.96 limits include = 95% of total observations
4. Mean ± 3SD limits include = 98.73% of total observations
5. Mean ± 2.58 SD limits include = 99% of total observations

In other words, in any normal distribution observation larger or smaller than Mean ± 1 SD covers only one third or 32% observations will lie outside the range.

Similarly, values more or less than ± 2SD are only 4.55% and values more or less than Mean ± 3SD are very rare and are only 0.27%

NORMAL CURVE

If we draw a frequency curve of the following observations of normal distribution table, the curve will have following characteristics:

– It is having one peak, so that mean, median, mode coincide.

– It is built up gradually from the smallest frequency at the extremes of classification to the highest frequency at the peak in the middle.

Characterstics

- It is symmetrical in nature
- It is bell shaped.
- It has no inflections. The central part is convex while at point of inflection the curve changes from convexity to concavity.
- A perpendicular from the point of inflection will cut the base at a distance of one SD from the mean on either side will include approximately 68% of the distribution values .

Z-SCORE

Deviation from mean in a normal distribution or a curve is called relative or standard normal deviation and is given the symbol Z.

The location of any element in a normal distribution can be expressed in terms of how many SDs' it lies below or above the mean (smaller or bigger than the mean) of the distribution and this is Z score of the element.

If element lies above the mean it will have +Z score and if element lies below the mean it will have –Z-score.

$$Z\text{-score} = \text{Element } -\text{Mean/ SD}$$
$$\text{i.e.} = \text{observation} - \text{Mean/SD}$$
$$= (x - \bar{x})/\text{SD}$$

Application of Z-Value

It allows us to calculate the probability of a score occuring within our normal distribution and enables us to compare two scores that are from different normal distribution.

Z–value states what proportion of any normal distribution lies above any given Z-value, e.g. if 0.3085 (approximately 31%) of any normal distribution has above a Z-value of 0.5 because normal distributions are symmetrical. This also means that 0.3085 of the distribution lies below a Z-value of –0.5. Therefore 31% of this population has a height below 157.5 cm.

- By subtracting the proportion from 1 it can be found 0.6915 or approximately 69% of the population is above 157.5 cm.
- Instead of using Z-score to find the proportion of a distribution corresponding to a particular score, the conversion can also be done by using Z- score to find the score that divide the distribution into specified proportions, for example if we want to

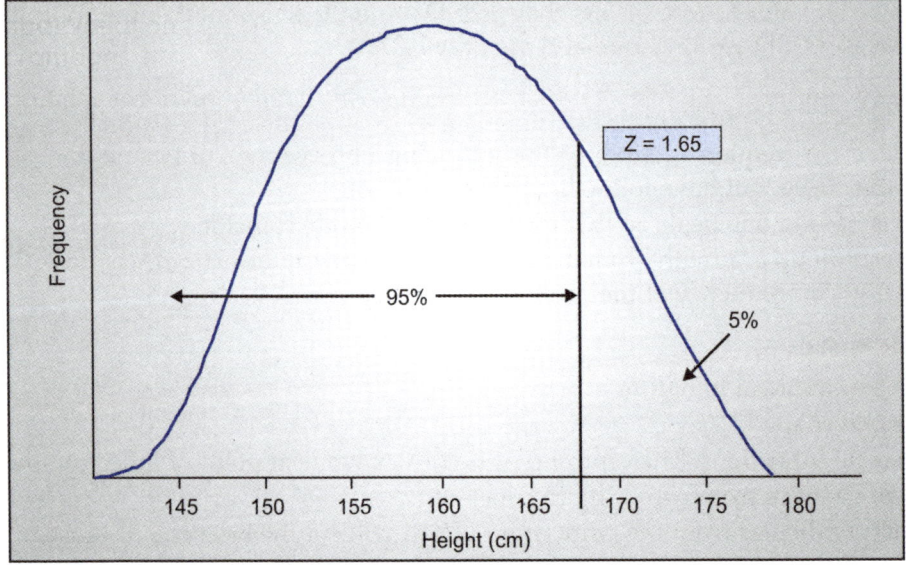

Fig. 16.2: Understanding of Z-value from a normal distribution curve

know what height divides the longest 5% of the population from the remaining 5%, we can use Z-score table.

The table shows that the Z-score corresponding to this approximate division (the nearest figure shown in the table is 0.495 rather than exactly 0.05) is 1.65

Thus, the corresponding height is 1.65 standard deviation above the mean, i.e. equal to mean + 1.65 SD, i.e. 160 +1.65 × 5 = 168.5

Table 16.2: Z-values

S. No	Z	Area beyond Z	Z	Area beyond Z
1	0.00	0.5000	1.65	0.0495
2	0.05	0.4801	1.70	0.0446
3	0.10	0.4602	1.75	0.0401
4	0.15	0.4404	1.80	0.0359
5	0.20	0.4207	1.85	0.0322
6	0.25	0.4013	1.90	0.0287
7	0.30	0.3821	1.95	0.0256
8	0.35	0.3632	2.00	0.0228
9	0.40	0.3446	2.05	0.0202
10	0.45	0.3264	2.10	0.0179
11	0.50	0.3085	2.15	0.0158
12	0.55	0.2912	2.20	0.0139
13	0.60	0.2743	2.25	0.0112
14	0.65	0.2578	2.30	0.0107
15	0.70	0.2420	2.35	0.0094
16	0.75	0.2266	2.40	0.0082
17	0.80	0.2119	2.45	0.0071
18	0.85	0.1977	2.50	0.0062
19	0.90	0.1841	2.55	0.0054
20	0.95	0.1711	2.60	0.0047
21	1.00	0.1587	2.65	0.0040
22	1.05	0.1469	2.70	0.0035
23	1.10	0.1357	2.75	0.0030
24	1.15	0.1251	2.80	0.0026
25	1.20	0.1151	2.85	0.0022
26	1.25	0.1056	2.90	0.0019
27	1.30	0.0968	2.95	0.0016
28	1.35	0.0885	3.00	0.0013
29	1.40	0.0808	3.05	0.0011
30	1.45	0.0735	3.10	0.0010
31	1.50	0.0668	3.15	0.0008
32	1.55	0.0606	3.20	0.0007
33	1.60	0.0548	3.30	0.0005

If Z for an observation height 165 cm is +1, i.e. it is one SD (5 cm) higher than mean (160 cm), it will cover 50% observations to the left of mean, $(x + 34\%)$ to the right of mean (as per normal distribution of observations), i.e. 84%. Only 16% of the total observations will lie above the value mean +1 SD. In other words, probability of having height above 165 cm is 16% or 0.16 out of one.

Similarly, if Z is 1.5SD (height 152.5 cm) only 8% $(100{-}50 - 34 - 8 = 8)$ people will have height below 152.5 cm.

In the standard normal curve the mean is taken as zero and SD as unity or one.

Example 1: Menstrual cycle in women following normal distribution has a mean of 28 days and SD of 2 days. How frequently would you expect a menstrual cycle (mc) of:
a. More than 30 Days?
b. Less than 22 Days?

Answer
a. As per normal distribution, 68% of the women will have a mc of mean +/− 1 SD, i.e. 28 ± 2 or 26 to 30 days, 32% will have longer or shorter mc. Because of symmetry in normal distribution, half the women, i.e. 16% women will have longer cycles, i.e. more than 30 days.

Or calculations may also be done as per unit normal distribution.

$$Z = (x - \bar{x})/SD = (30 - 28)/2 = 1$$

Referring to the table of unit normal distribution if $Z = 1$, the number of women in whom mc will exceed 30 days = 0.1587 out of one, i.e. 15.87%.

b. As per unit normal distribution

$$Z = (22 - 28)/2 = -6/2 = -3$$

Corresponding value as per the table is 0.0013; thus 0.13% women will have mc less than 22 days.

Example 2: Mean height of 500 students is 160 cm, the SD is 5 cm.
a. What are the chances of height above 175 cm, being normal if height follows normal distribution?
b. What percentage of boys will have heights above 168 cm?
c. How many of the boys will have heights between 168 and 175 cm?

Answer
a. $Z = (175{-}160)/5 = 15/5 = 3$

This corresponds to 0.0013 as per table of unit normal distribution. Thus only 0.13 of students will have height above 175 cm. The chances of being taller than 175 cm will be 0.13% only.

b. $Z = (168{-}160)/5 = 8/5 = 1.6$

This corresponds to 0.0548 as per table of unit normal distribution. Thus, number of boys above height of 168 cm. will be 5.48% only.

c. The number of boys having height above 168 cm. and below 175 will be 0.0548–0.0013= 0.0535 out of one. Thus, only 5.35% of students will have height with in range of 168–175 cm.

Example 3: The pulse rate of healthy males follow a normal distribution with a mean of 72/minute and a SD of 3.5/minute.

a. In what percentage of individuals, pulse rate will differ by 2 beats from the mean?
b. Mark out symmetrically around the mean, the range in which 50% of the individuals will lie?

Answer

a. $Z = (x - \bar{x})/SD = 74 - 72/\#.5 = 2/3.5 = 0.571$

Referring Z value 0.571 to the unit normal distribution table, the number of individuals in whom Pulse rate will exceed 74/minute will be 0.2843 out of 1 or 28.43%. Similarly, number that will have Pulse rate less than 70 per minute will be 28.43%. Thus, 28.43 + 28.43 = 56.86% of individuals the Pulse rate will differ by 2 beats from the Mean.

b. In the normal curve 34% individuals lie on either side of Mean up to 1 SD, i.e. 3.5 beats. So 25% will lie up to 3.5/34 × 25= 2.57

Make the area on both sides of mean up to 2.57/minute SD. Area thus marked will cover 25% + 25%= 50% of the individuals.

If a population's resting heart rate is normally distributed with a mean of 70 and standard deviation of 10, we can state what proportion of the population has a resting heart rate between certain limits.

Z-score also allowed us to specify the probability of a randomly picked element being above or below a particular score, e.g. if we know that 5% of population has a height more than 168.5 cm, then the probability of one randomly selected person from the population having a height above 168.5 cm will be 5% or 0.05.

As a ready reckoner, according to levels of significance these few Z-values with probability (P) can be recommended. These are as follows.

Z-value	1.6 (1.65)	2.0 (1.96)	2.3 (2.2)	2.6 (2.58)
P-value	0.1	0.05	0.02	0.01
Inference	Not significant	Significant	Significant	Highly significant

EXERCISES TO SOLVE

1. In one class, Rekha got 70 marks in one paper, while 100 is the mean of the class and SD is 15, then while getting 70 marks, where she stands, i.e. how many students are having more marks than Rekha.
2. Mean Hb of 100 girl students is 10 gm% with SD of 1.2. Calculate:
   i. What are the chances of Hb 11gm%, being normal if the Hb follows normal distribution?
   ii. What percentage of girls will have Hb above 12 gm%?
   iii. How many of the girls will have Hb between 11 and 12 gm%?
3. Systolic blood pressure of healthy males represent a normal distribution curve with mean 115 mmHg and SD 4.5 mmHg.

Calculate:
i. in what percentage of individuals, SBP will differ by 10 mmHg from the mean?
ii. mark out symmetrically, the range in which 50% of the individuals will be around the mean.

INTERPRETATION OF DATA

Knowledge of the application of statistical principles and methods is necessary not only for an understanding of biological and medical science, but also for effective practice in any of the health professions.

Because of variability in biological, clinical and laboratory data, knowledge of statistics is necessary and central to their understanding and interpretation.

It should be interpreted that there are some of the reasons, why it is necessary to interpret the data in a manner,

- To understand the rationale on which diagnostic, prognostic and therapeutic decisions are or should be based and that medicine is highly dependent on concepts of probability.
- To interpret laboratory tests, bed side observations and measurements in light of knowledge of physiology, observer and instrumental variations.
- To know and understand the statistical and epidemiological facts about etiology and prognosis of diseases treated in order to give best advice to patients about how to prevent or limit the effects of these diseases.
- To identify and describe the country's health problems and to utilize the resources available in the best possible manner.
- To develop crucial deductive faculties, which are needed throughout medical studies and thereafter in practice.

Statistics provides information support for health field. It is not an end in itself but is a means through which other disciplines may be better understood.

After analysis of data, observer or experimenter is actually interested in conclusions or to know the significance of differences he has observed.

PROBABILITY

It measures the relative frequency of a particular event happening by chance in the long run.

Inferences or conclusions drawn after various statistical analysis are based on theory of probability.

In a medical/health practice, what is the aim of the physician?

Whether the factor has a significant role in causation of disease or not? Whether the drug for a particular disease or a procedure applied in surgery is effective as treatment or not?

In normal distribution concept we have observed by knowing it as Mean $\pm$ SD We can interpret our findings as:

i. We can say – what is a probability of having a disease from a particular risk factor.
ii. or with how much confidence one can say about an event to occur.
iii. or what is the confidence limit of a physician or level of confidence in relation to interpretation of causal relationship.

Let us understand suppose a woman is pregnant. In this case the chance of getting male or female child is fifty-fifty. We can say—

   i. There are 50% chances to get male child.

  ii. Our level of confidence is 50% about the interpretation of event.

 iii. Our limit of predicting the event is 50%.

 iv. We have 50% chance to be false.

  v. Probability of finding the prediction true is 50%.

Take another case. In a married woman:

   i. Chance of having two successive male children is 25%.

  ii. Our level of confidence about the event to be true is 25%.

 iii. Probability of finding the prediction true is 25% and false is 75%.

Similarly, if there is a lucky draw and 1 out of ten is to get a prize, then there are only 10% chances for a person to get the prize. With confidence, we can say that there is no chance for 9 persons to win the prize.

If an event is to happen one out of 20, the chance or probability of happening reduces to 5%.

INTERPRETATION OF PROBABILITY

If an event is to occur one out of five it is not as significant as if it occur in case of one out of 20.

On the other hand, when an event is to occur one out of 100 and it happens to a person, it is very significant. So, in case of normal distribution, 95% confidence limit, i.e. (Mean $\pm$ 2 SD) or 5% probability of a particular event beyond the confidence limit is our own arbitrary line for significant or non-significant level.

Probability can be measured on a continuous scale of values between 0 and 1. An event that is impossible to occur, has a probability value of zero. An event that is certain to occur has a probability of occurrence equal to one.

If probability of an event happening is p and not happening is denoted by symbol q, then

$$p+q=1 \text{ or } p=1-q$$

Arithmetically p = Number of events occurred/Total number of trials

If twins are born over in 80 pregnancies then

$$p=1/80$$

STATISTICAL SIGNIFICANCE

At certain level of probability or confidence limit, which has been conventionally fixed by us, is that the likelihood of the result having occurred by chance is 0.5 or less. We can say it is significant and in the every day terminology – that it is important, noteworthy, or meaningful.

Suppose, a study comparing two types of drugs might conclude that one drug produced a statistically significant lower mean blood pressure than the other; but if it is a very minute difference, it would not be a substantively significant finding, and would not necessarily cause physicians to prescribe this drug rather than the other.

CONFIDENCE LIMIT

The limit of mean $\pm$ 1.96SD/SEs is called confidence limits, i.e. 95% confidence limit.

If an investigator wants to find the true mean pulse rate of large population, it would be impractical to take the pulse rate of every person in the population. Instead we can draw a random sample from the population and take a pulse of the people of sample provided the sample is truly random, the investigator can be 95% confident that the true population mean lies within $\pm$1.96SE of the sample mean obtained.

CONFIDENCE INTERVAL

The difference between the upper and lower confidence limits is called confidence interval.

Normally, researchers will want their confidence intervals to be as narrow as possible. The formula for confidence limit shows

$$\text{C.I.} = \text{Sample mean} \pm \text{Z-score}$$

Till now, we have discussed about population mean, population standard deviation, for which we require, normally distributed population.

But we see in practice that we are not having such data (population mean and population SD) for every kind of situation, e.g. generally whenever effectiveness of a new drug or a surgical procedure is to be predicted, it has been tested on only a small sample of patients.

As it is not always possible to cover an entire population under a study, most of the investigations are carried out on sample basis. However, it is unlikely that a sample will be a true representative of the population from which it is drawn. It will not exactly reflect its corresponding population mean. If it cannot be expected to be exactly same, there will be sampling error that will cause the sample statistic to differ from population statistics.

However, if a series of samples are taken from the same population, their values are bound to differ to a certain extent. If more and more samples are taken from the population and their values are presented in a frequency distribution table, it shall constitute a Sampling Distribution Series.

The standard deviation of the random sampling distribution of mean, has its own name the standard error or standard error of the mean.

STANDARD ERROR

It is the SD of random sample distribution of means, has its own name SE or SEM.

It is a measure of the extent to which the sample mean deviates from the true population mean.

$$SE = \frac{\text{Pop.SD}}{\sqrt{n}} = \frac{\text{SD of the given population}}{\sqrt{\text{Size of sample}}}$$

SE is inversely proportional to size of sample, which means larger the sample, more closely will the sample mean represent the true population mean.

So, it is due to this reason that surveys of large sample size are more trusted.

Standard Error is the Value

1. That defines the confidence limits of population mean.

2. Comparison of SE values of two samples drawn from the same population can decide whether the difference between the two is significant or not, i.e.
   - Comparison of experiment or control group
   - Observations before and after an exposure
   - Basis for the application of t-test

3. To study the significance of variability between the means or proportions of two large samples and between means or proportions of population as a whole and a sample drawn from it.

4. The significance of difference between the means of two samples drawn from same population or two groups drawn from two different populations.

17

Test of Significance

A test of significance is a process by which we gather evidence as to how far the sample value matches the population value.

In these tests, first we formulate a **Null Hypothesis**. We assume that the factor under study has no effect and the observed difference is entirely due to chance. In hypothesis testing, the null hypothesis is either accepted or rejected, depending upon whether the p-value is above or below a pre-determined cut-off point, known as significance level of test. The different formulae used to calculate probability that the differences those found in the observed data have occurred by chance. This calculated value of probability is known as p-value.

If p-value is low, it indicates that differences occurred by chance in a small proportion of all possible samples. This is taken as evidence that it is unlikely (although still possible) that the observed results arose from chance alone.

If p-value is high, it indicates that differences observed would occur by chance in high proportion of possible samples, even if there were no differences in the underlying population.

If p-value is less than cut-off point, null hypothesis rejected.

If p-value is greater than or equal to cut-off point, null hypothesis is accepted.

It is usual to choose 0.05 (5%) or 0.01 (1%) as significance level for testing the null hypothesis.

Note
- The test never serve as a proof.
- The test give no information about the cause of difference, beyond stating the probability of chance operating.
- The test cannot correct the mistake in collection of data and experimental design.

There are following tests of significance:

For quantitative data
1. Coefficient of variation
2. Standard error of mean
3. Standard error of difference between two means

- Z-test, if sample is large
- t-test, if sample is small

4. Karl–Pearson coefficient for correlation
5. Anova test

For Qualitative Data

1. Standard error of proportion
2. Standard error of difference between two proportion
   - Z-test, if sample is large
   - Chi-square test, if sample is small
3. Spearman's rank formula for correlation

TESTS FOR QUANTITATIVE DATA

1. Coefficient of Variation

This test is used to overcome the limitation of SD. It is a measure used to compare relative variability. The variation of the same character in two or more different series has to be compared often, e.g. height or weight of Punjabis and Tamils. On the other hand variation of two different characters in one and the same series has to be compared just as height and weight, blood pressure and weight or blood pressure and pulse rate.

$$CV = \frac{SD}{Mean} \times 100$$

2. Standard Error of Mean

It is the difference between the mean of observed values from a sample and mean value of universe or population measured by statistics, it measures the chance of variation between sample and universe.

$$SE\bar{x} = \frac{SD}{\sqrt{n}} = \text{Standard deviation} \times \sqrt{\text{Total number of persons in the sample}}$$

Example: The mean Hb value of 100 women was 10 gm% with SD of 1.5. The mean Hb of women in Patiala is 11 gm%. Is the difference between the two by chance?

$$SE\bar{x} = \frac{SD}{\sqrt{n}} = \frac{1.5}{10} = 0.15$$

Interpretation

Considering cut off point at 95%, confidence limit (mean ± 2SD) of the mean Hb of women in Patiala, i.e.

11 + (2 × 0.15) to 11 – (2 × 0.15)

It is 11.3 – 10.7 gm%

Inference

Since, 10 gm% is outside the range, null hypothesis is rejected, i.e. the variation may be by chance and there might be other factors.

Thus, we say that the difference is significant.

Uses

- To work out the desired confidence limits within which the population mean would lie.
- To determine whether the sample is drawn from a known population or not, when its mean is known.
- To find SE of difference between two means to know if the observed difference between the means of two samples is real and statistically significant.
- To calculate the minimum size of sample, in order to have desired confidence limit, if SD of population is known.

3. Standard Error of Difference between two Means

If two independent, large and random samples are drawn in pairs, repeatedly from the same population and each time the difference between the means of two samples is calculated it is the standard error of difference between the two means, from which we will know whether the difference is by chance or not.

Uses

1. Means of normally distributed variables in the two similar or different groups can be compared such as height, weight, blood pressure, pulse rate, etc.
2. The action of a drug on a variable such as BP or pulse rate is compared in two groups, when a placebo is given in the control group and drug in the other group.
3. The action of two different drugs or two different doses of same drug can be compared.

Z-TEST

If the sample is larger than 30, Z-test is applied.

Calculations

$$SE\left(\bar{x}_1 - \bar{x}_2\right) = \sqrt{\frac{(SD_1)^2}{\sqrt{n_1}} + \frac{(SD_2)^2}{\sqrt{n_2}}}$$

$$Z\text{-value} = \frac{\text{Observed difference between two sample means}}{\text{Standard error of difference between two means}}$$

Example:

There are two groups of 100 and 150 children each. Mean height of group one is 60 cm and second group is 62 cm. The SD is 2.5 cm and 3 cm respectively. Is this difference statistically significant?

$$SE\left(\bar{x}_1 - \bar{x}_2\right) = \sqrt{\frac{(SD_1)^2}{\sqrt{n_1}} + \frac{(SD_2)^2}{\sqrt{n_2}}}$$

$$= \sqrt{\frac{(2.5)^2}{100} + \frac{(3.0)^2}{150}} = 0.35$$

$$Z\text{-value} = \frac{60 - 62}{0.35} = 5.71$$

If the difference between two samples (groups of children) is significant, then the value should be beyond 95% confidence limit, i.e. $2 \times SE = 2 \times 0.35 = 0.7$. But here it is even more than 3 SE, i.e. $3 \times 0.35 = 1.05$.

Inference

The observed difference as calculated is more than 3 times the SE and hence, it is highly significant. The growth is more in second group than in the first.

STUDENT'S t-TEST

If the sample size is small, then student's t-test is applied.

It is applied to find the significance of difference between two means as

(I) unpaired t-test   (II) Paired t-test

I. Unpaired t-test

Criteria for application
- Random samples
- Quantitative data
- Variable–normally distributed
- Sample size <30

Steps of calculation
- Write observations
- Square them
- Add them individually
- Find the mean
- Calculate combined SD

$$SD = \sqrt{\sum x_1^2 - \frac{\left(\sum x_1^2\right)}{n_1} + \sum x_2^2 - \frac{\left(\sum x_2^2\right)}{n_2}}$$

- Calculate SE

$$SE = SD \times \sqrt{\frac{1}{n_1} + \frac{1}{n_2}}$$

- Calculate t-value

$$t = \frac{\text{Difference of mean}}{SE}$$

- Calculate degree of freedom: $df = n_1 + n_2 - 2$

Example:

In a nutritional study, 13 children were given a usual diet plus vitamin A and D tablets while the second comparable group of 12 children was taking the usual diet. After a year the gain in weight in kilograms was noted which is given in Table 17.1.

Can we say that vitamin A and D were responsible for this difference?

Table 17.1: Calculation of unpaired t-test

Group I		Group II	
(x_1)	$(x_1)^2$	(x_2)	$(x_2)^2$
5	25	1	1
3	9	3	9
4	16	2	4
3	9	4	16
2	4	2	4
6	36	1	1
3	9	3	9
2	4	4	16
3	9	3	9
6	36	2	4
7	49	2	4
5	25	2	4
3	9	3	9
Total 52	240	30	86

Mean (Group I) = 52/13 = 4: Mean (Group II) = 30/12 = 2.5

$$SD = \sqrt{\sum x_1^2 - \frac{\left(\sum x_1^2\right)}{n_1} + \Sigma x_2^2 - \frac{\left(\sum x_2^2\right)}{n_2}}$$

$$= \sqrt{240 - \frac{(52)^2}{13} + 86 - \frac{(30)^2}{12}} = 6.6$$

$$SE = SD \times \sqrt{\frac{1}{n_1} + \frac{1}{n_2}} = 6.6 \times \sqrt{\frac{1}{13} + \frac{1}{12}} = 2.7$$

$$t = \frac{4 - 2.5}{2.7} = 0.58$$

$$df = 13 + 12 - 2 = 23$$

Now refer to t-table and find the t-value corresponding to the degree of freedom of 23 at the cut-off point of 0.05.

This value in the t-table is 2.07.

Here the value is less, so the difference is insignificant.

II. Paired t-test

It is applied to paired test of independent observations. From one sample only, when each individual gives a pair or two observations, e.g.

- If we want to know role of a factor when the observations are made before and after it play, e.g. of exertion on pulse rate; of a drug on BP
- To compare effect of two drugs given to same individual at two different occasions, e.g. adrenaline and nor-adrenaline.

- To compare the accuracy of two different instruments.
- To compare results of two different lab techniques, e.g. estimation of Hb by Tallquist and Sahli's method.
- To compare observations made at two different sites in the body of the same person, e.g. temperature in maxilla and mouth of the same individual.

As per null hypothesis, it is assumed that there is no real difference between the Mean, before and after observations.

Steps of Calculation

- Write observations
- Find the difference
- Square the difference
- Add both individually
- Calculate combined SD

$$SD = \sqrt{\frac{\sum dx^2 - \frac{(\sum dx)^2}{n}}{n-1}}$$

- Calculate SE

$$SE = \frac{SD}{\sqrt{n}}$$

- Calculate t-value
- Calculate df, i.e $n-1$

Example:

In a group of hypertensive individuals, systolic blood pressure was noted before and after the administration of an antihypertensive drug. Has the administered drug lowered the BP?

Table 17.2: Calculation of paired t-test

Before Drug	After Drug	Difference dx	Squared dx²
122	120	2	4
121	118	3	9
120	115	5	25
115	110	5	25
126	122	4	16
130	130	0	0
120	116	4	16
125	124	1	1
128	125	3	9
		$\Sigma dx = 27$	$\Sigma dx^2 = 105$

∴ Mean $= 27/9 = 3$

$$SD = \sqrt{\frac{105 - \frac{(27)^2}{9}}{9-1}} = 1.73$$

$$SE = \frac{1.73}{\sqrt{9-1}} = 0.58$$

t = Difference between mean/SE = 3/0.58 = 5.17

$$df = n - 1 \text{ or } 9 - 1 = 8$$

Now refer to t-table and find calculated *t*-value corresponding to the degree of freedom of 8 at the cut-off point of 0.05.

This value in the table is 2.31.

The observed value is more than this. So, there is no doubt that drug has produced the effect.

So, we can interpret it as t-value = 5.17, df = 8, P < 0.001, highly significant.

EXERCISES TO SOLVE

1. In a universe, the average number of attacks of common cold was 4.5 per person with a SD of 2.87. A sample of 20 persons drawn from the same universe showed the number of attacks of cold per person as follows…

   7, 2, 5, 0, 1   5, 5, 6, 7, 6   2, 6, 9, 4, 8   8, 6, 7, 9, 3

   i. Calculate the mean, SD and SE of the mean
   ii. Comment why SD and SE of mean are different?
   iii. Give 95% confidence limits of attacks of common cold in universe and examine whether all these observations in the sample lie within the confidence limits or not.

2. Serum protein is lower in females than in males. Justify this conclusion by applying appropriate statistical technique to the data given below:

Sex	Number (n)	Mean serum protein level in gm/100 ml	SD
Male	18	7.21	0.26
Female	7	6.90	1.28

3. Chest circumference in cm of 10 normal children and 10 malnourished children aged 1 year are given below. Normal group: 42, 46, 50, 48, 50, 52, 41, 49, 51 and 56. Malnourished group: 38, 41, 36, 35, 30, 42, 31, 29, 31, 35. Test for the statistical significance of the difference in chest circumference, on an average between these two groups.

4. A group of 15 normal children in a study had a mean bilirubin level of 1.05 µ% and SD of 0.34. Another group of 15 children with infantile cirrhosis of liver had mean bilirubin level of 4.99 µ% and SD of 2.52. Is the difference between the 2 means statistically significant?

5. The systolic blood pressure of 6 hypertensive patients were 179,190,183,165,180, and 175 mm of Hg. After administration of a particular drug for 1 week the pressures were 175,180,187,150,170 and 180 mm of Hg respectively. Could such differences arise due to chance?

TEST FOR QUALITATIVE DATA

Standard Error of Proportion

It is defined as a unit that measures variation of an attribute, which occurs in the proportions of a character attribute from sample to sample or from population to sample in a qualitative data.

It is of particular importance in medical statistics and is frequently used to find the efficacy of

- a drug
- a line of treatment
- a vaccine
- operation
- the part played by other causal factors

$$SEP = p \times q/n$$

p = percentage of positive character

q = percentage of alternate character

n = number of sample

Uses and Application

1. To find confidence limits of sample proportion when population proportion is known.
2. To determine whether the sample is drawn from the known population or not when the proportion in population is known.
3. To find standard error of difference between two proportions to know whether the observed difference is statistically significant or it is apparent and insignificant and due to chance.
4. To find the minimum size of sample, if the population proportion is known.

Example

I : Polymorph count was 350 out of 500 W.B.C. At 95% confidence limit, within what limits the population proportion will lie?

$$p = 350/500 \times 100 = 70$$

$$q = 100 - 70 = 30$$

$$SEP = \sqrt{\frac{p \times q}{n}} = \sqrt{\frac{70 \times 30}{500}} = 2.05$$

At 95% confidence limit

$$70 \pm 2 \; SEP = 70 \pm 2 \times 2.05 = 70 \pm 4.1$$

i.e. 65.9–74.1

II : In a village of Punjab, 80% persons are suffering from gingivitis. A study of 200 persons showed that 75% persons were suffering from gingivitis. Is this difference by chance or statistically significant.

$$p = 80\%$$
$$q = 100 - 80 = 20\%$$
$$n = 200$$

$$\text{SEP} = \sqrt{\frac{P \times q}{n}} = \sqrt{\frac{80 \times 20}{200}} = 2.83$$

At 95% confidence limit: $80 \pm 2\ \text{SE} = 80 \pm 2 \times 2.83$

i.e. $74.34 - 85.66$

Inference

In a sample 75% lies between $74.34 - 85.66$ range, the study sample is likely to be from the same village and the difference is not statistically significant.

III: What should be the size of sample for assessing prevalence rate of oral cancer in an urban population where the prevalence was given as 3% in the age group above 15 years. Allowable error is 10% of positive character with 5% risk.

$$\text{SEP} = \sqrt{\frac{p \times q}{n}} \quad \text{at 95\% limit SEP} = \sqrt{\frac{p \times q}{n}}$$

$$(\text{SEP})^2 = 4 \times \frac{p \times q}{n}$$

$$n = 4 \times \frac{p \times q}{(\text{S.E.P.})^2}$$

SEP = $10/100 \times 3 = 0.3$ with 95% of confidence limit or 5% risk factor.

$$n = 4 \times \frac{3 \times 97}{0.3 \times 0.3} = 12933$$

Standard Error of Difference between two Proportions

The differences in the pairs of proportion or percentages of samples drawn from the same population are also normally distributed, i. e. standard error of difference between two means.

The same Z-test is applied.

SE $(p_1 - p_2)$ is calculated as

$$\sqrt{\frac{p_1 q_1}{n_1} + \frac{p_2 q_2}{n_2}}$$

Z-value = Observed difference/SE $(p_1 - p_2)$

In actual practice, we do not know the value of population proportion and we have only two samples. So we have to substitute the value noticed in one sample in place of P and compare it with that of other sample.

Such a substitution is valid, if the samples are large and drawn at random.

If Z-value is > 2: It is significant at 95% confidence limit, i.e. in 95% cases it would not happen by chance. The chance of its being normal are only 5%. The difference is abnormal or real and may be due to influence of some external factor.

If Z value is > 3 then it is significant at 99% of confidence limit, i.e. highly significant.

Example

A-vaccine was given to 90 children and B-vaccine was given to 86 children. During the attack of disease, 22 and 14 children respectively had the disease. Is the difference in efficacy of vaccines statistically significant (Table 17.3)?

Table 17.3: Calculation for Z-test

Type	Vaccine given	Disease	Attack Rate
A	90	22	$22/90 \times 100 = 24.4\%$
B	86	14	$14/86 \times 100 = 16.2\%$

p for A = 24.4% $q = 100 - 24.4\% = 75.6\%$
p for B = 16.2% $q = 100 - 16.2\% = 83.8\%$

$$SE = \sqrt{\frac{p_1 q_1}{n_1} + \frac{p_2 q_2}{n_2}} = \sqrt{\frac{24.4 \times 75.6}{90} + \frac{16.2 \times 83.8}{86}} = 6.02$$

Observed difference = 24.4 – 16.2 = 8.2

   Z value = 8.2/6.02 = 1.3

So, the Z-value is less than 2, the critical value at the level of significance, i.e. 95% confidence limit. So the difference is insignificant.

CHI-SQUARE TEST : χ^2-TEST

- It is used in qualitative data when the size of sample is small.
- It is very useful in this respect and is most commonly used when data is in frequencies such as the number of responses in two or more categories.
- It can be used with any data, which can be reduced to proportions or percentages.
- It can be used in binomial samples, i.e. vaccinated vs. unvaccinated, died vs survived and also for multinomial samples like socio-economic class I, II, III, IV, illiterate, primary, matric, graduate, etc.
- It can also be used for finding association between two events, i.e. smoking and cancer, weight and diabetes.

Essentials to Apply Chi-square Test

- A random sample
- Qualitative data
- Lowest observed frequency not less than 5

Calculation of χ^2 Test

$$\chi^2 = \frac{\sum (O - E)^2}{E}$$

$$\text{Chi-square} = \frac{\text{Sum (Total) of (Mean observed frequency} - \text{Mean expected frequency)}^2}{\text{Mean expected frequency}}$$

Example

The outcome of treatment with drug and placebo among experimental and control group is given in Table 17.4:

Table 17.4: Calculation for chi-square test

Group	Outcome		Total
	Dead	Survived	
Control	10	25	35
Experiment	5	60	65
Total	15	85	100

Steps to calculate

$$E = \frac{\text{Total no. of column (vertical)} \times \text{Total no. of row (horizontal)}}{\text{Grand total}}$$

$O = 10,$ $\qquad E = \dfrac{15 \times 35}{100} = 5.25$

$O = 25,$ $\qquad E = \dfrac{35 \times 85}{100} = 29.75$

$O = 5,$ $\qquad E = \dfrac{15 \times 65}{100} = 9.75$

$O = 60,$ $\qquad E = \dfrac{65 \times 85}{100} = 55.25$

χ^2 for each cell:

$O = 10,$ $\qquad \dfrac{(O-E)^2}{E} = \dfrac{(10-5.25)^2}{5.25} = 4.29$

$O = 25,$ $\qquad = \dfrac{(25-29.75)^2}{29.75} = 0.75$

$O = 5,$ $\qquad = \dfrac{(5-9.75)^2}{9.75} = 2.31$

$O = 60,$ $\qquad = \dfrac{(60-55.25)^2}{55.25} = 0.4$

Total χ^2 value $= 4.29 + 0.75 + 2.3 + 0.4 = 7.77$

To calculate df : $\qquad (c-1)(r-1) = (2-1)(2-1) = 1 \times 1 = 1$

On referring χ^2 table at 1 df the value of χ^2 under probability 0.05 is 3.84

Here the chi-square value is 7.77 which is higher than 3.84. Hence the result is significant. The drug has played its role in lowering the mortality.

So it is written as: $\chi^2 = 7.77$, df $= 1$, $p < 0.05$

ANOVA TEST (VARIANCE RATIO TEST)

Anova Test (Variance Ratio Test): This test involves another distribution called F-distribution:

Most of the time it is confined to comparing two samples means, but more than two samples drawn from corresponding normal populations can also be compared.

Suppose you want to know whether occupation plays any part in causation of high blood pressure? Record BP of 10 officers, 10 clerks, and 10 randomly selected lab technicians and 10 attendants.

Find mean and SD (variances) of BP of these four classes of employees.

If occupation plays no role in the causation of BP, the 4 groups when compared among them will not differ significantly. If occupation is playing a significant role, then 4 means will differ significantly.

To test whether the four means differ significantly or not, F-test or analysis of variance test has to be applied.

We start with null hypothesis that BP is independent of occupation.

We proceed as follows:

Steps:

1. Calculate sum of all
2. Calculate mean of each series
3. Square the sum of all series
4. Split this into two components
   a. Sum of squares between the series
   b. Sum of squares within the series
   Sum of squares = Total sum of squares of entire sample – Sum of squares between the class within class/series
5. Calculate df
6. Calculate F-ratio
7. Compare calculated F-ratio with F-table at df between the series and df within the series at 5% level of significance.

Example: Calculation for Anova test is shown is Table 17.5.

Table 17.5: Calculation for Anova test

	Officers	Clerks	Lab tech.	Attendants
	125	120	120	118
	130	122	115	120
	135	115	115	118
	120	110	130	120
	115	125	120	120
	120	122	125	115
	130	120	122	125
	135	120	115	125
	140	126	126	120
	135	120	118	115
Total	1285	1200	1206	1196
Mean	128.5	120	120.6	119.6

$\therefore$ Mean = 1285 + 1200 + 1206 + 1196 = 4887

$(\Sigma x)^2$ of all observations $= (125)^2 + (130)^2 + (135)^2 + \ldots + (115)^2 = 598751$

Total sum of square within class $= \sum x^2 - \dfrac{\left(\sum x\right)^2}{n} = 598751 - \dfrac{(4887)^2}{40} = 1681.7$

Sum of square between classes

$$= \frac{\left(\sum x_1\right)^2}{n_1} + \frac{\left(\sum x_2\right)^2}{n_2} + \frac{\left(\sum x_3\right)^2}{n_3} + \frac{\left(\sum x_4\right)^2}{n_4} + L\ L + \frac{\left(\sum x_n\right)^2}{N}$$

$$= \frac{(1285)^2}{10} + \frac{(1200)^2}{10} + \frac{(1206)^2}{10} + \frac{(1196)^2}{10} + L\ L + \frac{(4887)^2}{40} = 538.4$$

Error sum of squares = total sum of squares – occupation sum of squares.
Anova table (Table 17.6).

Table 17.6: Calculation of F-ratio

Sum of variance	df	Sum of squares	Mean sum of squares	F-ratio
a. Between occupation	$4 - 1 = 3$	538.48	$538.4/3 = 179.4$	$179.4/31.76 = 5.65$
b. Error	$39 - 3 = 36$	1143.3	$1143.3/36 = 31.76$	
Total	$40 - 1 = 39$	1681.78		

Now consult/refer to F-table for df 3 across and df 36 vertically at 5% level of significance.

This value in Table 17.6 is 2.86.

Since, computed F-ratio is more than table value (critical value) the mean BP differs significantly.

CORRELATION AND REGRESSION

We as a physician, a biostatistician, usually need to establish if there is a relationship between two characteristics, i.e. high temperature and pulse rate, height and weight, people's salt intake and their blood pressure or between the number of cigarettes smoke and their life expectancy.

The methods used to know this is correlation techniques. There are two basic kinds of correlation techniques:

- Correlation
- Regression

Correlation is used to establish and quantify the STRENGTH and DIRECTION of the relationship between two variables. Regression is used to express the Functional Relationship between two variables, so that the value of one can be predicted from the knowledge of the other.

Correlation

A correlation simply expresses the strength and direction of the relationship between two variables in terms of a correlation coefficient. Value of correlation coefficient vary from -1 to $+1$.

The strength of relationship is indicated by—size of coefficient.

The direction is indicated by—sign (plus or minus)

+ ve sign = positive correlation, e.g. high salt intake and high B.P

– ve sign = negative correlation, e.g high cigarettes low life expectancy

+1 or –1—perfect linear relationship

Zero — absolutely no relationship

> ± 0.5 — regarded as strong correlation

0 ± 0.5 — regarded as weak correlation

The relationship between two variables being correlated forms a bivariate distribution, which is commonly presented graphically in the form of a scatter graph.

First variable says height is usually plotted on the horizontal (X), whereas the second variable says weight is plotted on the vertical (Y) axis. There is likelihood of 4 types of diagrams (Fig. 17.1).

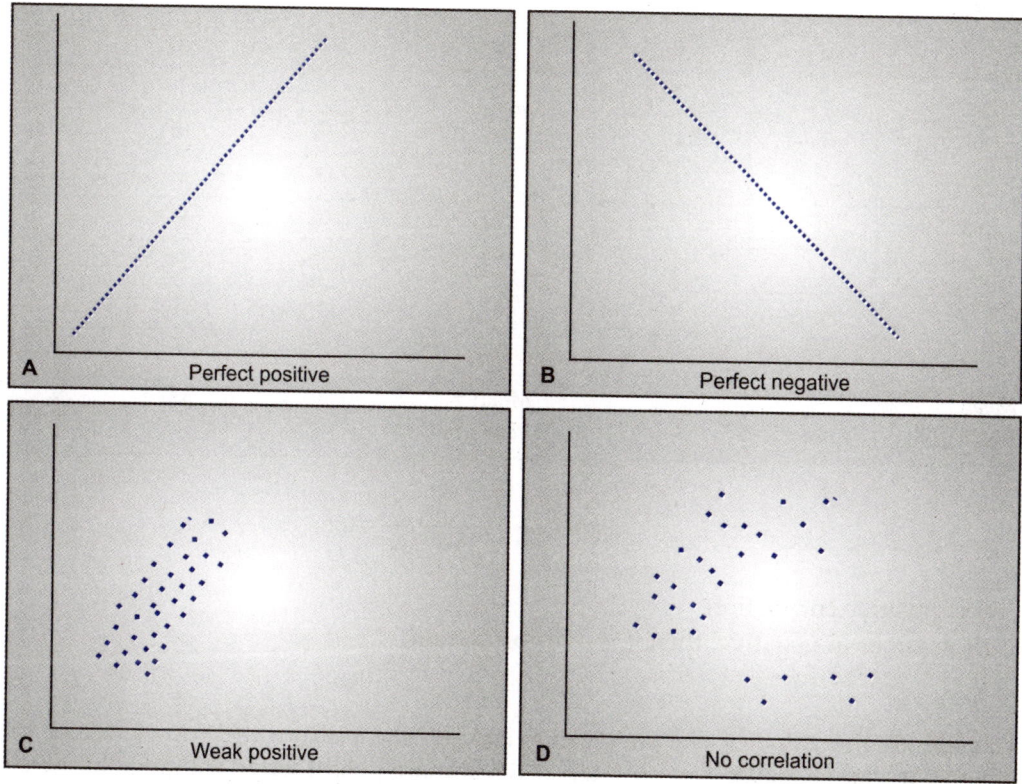

Fig. 17.1: Various types of correlation (A – D)

Types of correlation coefficient:

The two most commonly used correlation coefficients are:

- *Pearson product-moment correlation*
  It is used for quantitative data or ratio scale data.
  It is symbolized by 'r'.
- *Spearman rank-order correlation*
  It is used for qualitative data or ordinal scale data.
  It is symbolized by 'ρ' (rho).

Calculation of Correlation Coefficient

It is obtained by dividing products of corresponding deviations of various items from their means by product of their SDs and number of pairs of observations

$$r = \frac{\sum (x - \bar{x})(y - \bar{y})}{\sqrt{(x - \bar{x})^2 \sum (y - \bar{y})^2}} = \frac{\sum dd'}{\sqrt{\sum d^2 d'^2}}$$

Example:

Correlation between the heights of 8 fathers and their 8 sons (Table 17.7).

Table 17.7: Calculation of correlation coefficient

Height of father x	$x - \bar{x}$ d	$(x - \bar{x})^2$ d^2	Height of son y	$y - \bar{y}$ d	$(y - \bar{y})^2$ d'^2	dd'
65	−3	9	67	−2	4	6
66	−2	4	68	−1	1	2
67	−1	1	65	−4	16	4
67	−1	1	68	−1	1	1
68	0	0	72	+3	9	0
69	+1	1	72	+3	9	3
70	+2	4	69	0	0	0
71	+3	9	71	+2	4	6
Mean = 544/8 = 68		29	**Mean =** 552/8 = 69		44	22

$$r = \frac{\sum dd'}{\sqrt{\sum d^2 d'^2}} = \frac{22}{\sqrt{29 \times 44}} = 0.6$$

It is positive correlation.

(If it comes in negative, then it is −ve correlation).

Regression

To estimate the value of one character (variable, say y) from the knowledge of the other character (variable, say x), such as to estimate height when weight is known.

This is possible when the two are linearly correlated.

The former variable (y, i.e. weight) to be estimated is called dependent variable and later (x, i.e. height) which is known is called the independent variable.

This is done by finding regression coefficient.

Regression means change in the measurement of a variable character, on the positive or negative side, beyond the mean.

Calculation of regression coefficient (b)

Regression coefficient of y on x is denoted by b_{yx}

$$b_{yx} = \frac{\text{SD of } y \text{ series}}{\text{SD of } x \text{ series}} \times r \text{ (coefficient of correlation)}$$

If means are already calculated, then

$$b_{yx} = \frac{\sum dd'}{\sum d^2}$$

EXERCISES TO SOLVE

1. In order to determine the effect of certain OCP on weight gain, 9 healthy females were weighed prior to the start of its use and again at the end of a 3 months period.

Subject no.	Initial weight in kg	Weight after 3 months
1	48	49.2
2	56.4	57.2
3	52.0	56.0
4	60.0	58.0
5	54.0	56.0
6	56.0	57.2
7	48.0	47.2
8	56.0	56.4
9	52.0	52.8

Is there a sufficient evidence to conclude that females experienced gain in weight following 3 months of the OCP use.

2. In a screw manufacturing industry, out of 120 untrained workers 36 were injured during work while out of 80 trained workers 8 were injured in the same period of time. Justify the role of training.

3. A survey of 400 children in age group 0–5 years showed prevelance rate of protein calorie malnutrition to be 15%. Another study showed a prevalence of 5% in a sample of 300 of similar age group. Can we say that there is a statistical significance in the difference between the 2 prevalence rates?

4. Determine if there is any association between scabies amongst the school children and the socio-economic status of their parents (Table 17.8).

Table 17.8: Socio-economic status

Scabies status	1	2	3	4	5	Total
No. of children with scabies	23	127	640	806	63	1659
No. of children without scabies	427	1573	7560	7526	541	17627
Total	450	1700	8200	8332	604	19286

5. Does the following data suggest any association between the educational status of mothers and their belief about the child's topfeed needs?

EDUCATION STATUS OF MOTHERS

Top feeding belief	Illiterate school	Primary school	Middle school	High school	University	Total
Yes	2	24	25	34	10	96
No	3	6	4	2	0	15
Total	5	30	29	36	10	111

Annexures

Table of 't'*

df	0.10	0.05	0.02	0.01	0.001
1	6.31	12.71	3.82	63.662	636.62
2	2.92	4.30	6.97	9.93	31.60
3	2.35	3.18	4.54	5.84	12.92
4	2.13	2.78	3.75	4.60	8.61
5	2.02	2.57	3.37	4.03	6.87
6	1.94	2.45	3.14	3.71	5.96
7	1.90	2.37	3.00	3.50	5.41
8	1.86	2.31	2.90	3.36	5.04
9	1.83	2.26	2.82	3.25	4.78
10	1.81	2.23	2.76	3.17	4.59
11	1.80	2.20	2.72	3.11	4.44
12	1.78	2.18	2.68	3.06	4.32
13	1.77	2.16	2.65	3.01	4.22
14	1.76	2.15	2.62	2.98	4.14
15	1.75	2.13	2.60	2.95	4.07
16	1.75	2.12	2.58	2.92	4.02
17	1.74	2.11	2.57	2.90	3.97
18	1.73	2.10	2.55	2.88	3.92

(Contd.)

(*Contd.*)

Table of 't'*				
19	1.73	2.09	2.54	2.86	3.88
20	1.73	2.09	2.53	2.85	3.85
21	1.72	2.08	2.52	2.83	3.82
22	1.72	2.07	2.51	2.82	3.79
23	1.71	2.07	2.50	2.81	3.77
24	1.71	2.06	2.49	2.80	3.75
25	1.71	2.06	2.49	2.79	3.73
26	1.71	2.06	2.48	2.78	3.71
27	1.70	2.05	2.47	2.77	3.69
28	1.70	2.05	2.47	2.76	3.67
29	1.70	2.05	2.46	2.76	3.66
30	1.69	2.04	2.46	2.75	3.65
40	1.68	2.02	2.42	2.70	3.55
60	1.67	2.00	2.39	2.66	3.46
120	1.66	1.98	2.36	2.62	3.37
infinity	1.65	1.96	2.33	2.58	3.29

*The table gives the probability of observing the highest 't' value by chance at particular degree of freedom. The probability of observing value of 't' greater than 2.95 at 15 degrees of freedom is 0.01 or 1%

ANNEXURE – B

Table of χ^2-square, Probability (p)*

df	0.50	0.10	0.05	0.02	0.01	0.001
1	0.46	2.71	3.84	5.41	6.64	10.83
2	1.39	4.61	5.99	7.82	9.21	13.82
3	2.37	6.25	7.82	9.84	11.34	16.27
4	3.36	7.78	9.49	11.67	13.28	18.47
5	4.35	9.24	11.07	13.39	15.09	20.52
6	5.35	10.65	12.59	15.03	16.81	22.46
7	6.35	12.02	14.07	16.62	18.48	24.32
8	7.34	13.36	15.51	18.17	20.09	16.13
9	8.34	14.68	16.92	19.68	21.67	27.88
10	9.34	15.89	18.31	21.16	23.21	29.59
11	10.34	17.28	19.68	22.62	24.73	31.26
12	11.34	18.55	21.03	24.05	26.22	32.91
13	12.34	19.81	22.36	25.47	27.69	34.53
14	13.34	21.06	23.69	26.87	29.14	36.12
15	14.34	22.31	24.99	28.26	30.58	37.70
16	15.34	23.54	26.30	29.63	32.00	39.25
17	16.34	24.77	27.59	30.99	33.41	40.79
18	17.34	25.99	28.87	32.35	34.81	42.31
19	18.34	27.20	30.14	33.69	36.19	42.82
20	19.34	28.41	31.41	35.02	37.57	45.32
21	20.34	29.62	32.67	36.34	38.93	46.80
22	21.34	30.81	33.92	37.66	40.29	48.27
23	22.34	32.01	35.17	38.97	41.64	49.73
24	23.34	33.20	36.42	40.27	42.98	51.18
25	24.34	34.38	37.65	41.57	44.31	52.62
26	25.34	35.56	38.89	42.86	45.64	54.05
27	26.34	36.74	40.11	44.14	46.96	55.48
28	27.34	37.92	41.34	45.42	48.28	56.89
29	28.34	39.09	42.56	46.69	49.59	58.30
30	29.34	40.26	43.77	47.96	50.89	59.70

* The table gives the highest value of chi square, at particular degrees of freedom, corresponding to probability P of occurrence by chance in nature, e.g. at 10 degrees of freedom chi square value larger than 18.31 will occur less than 5 times in 100 (P<0.05) and is interpreted as significance at 5% level.

Index

Reader's Notes

Reader's Notes

Reader's Notes